SJANIE HUGO BA, D.HYP, PGD.HYP, GHR, MBSCH

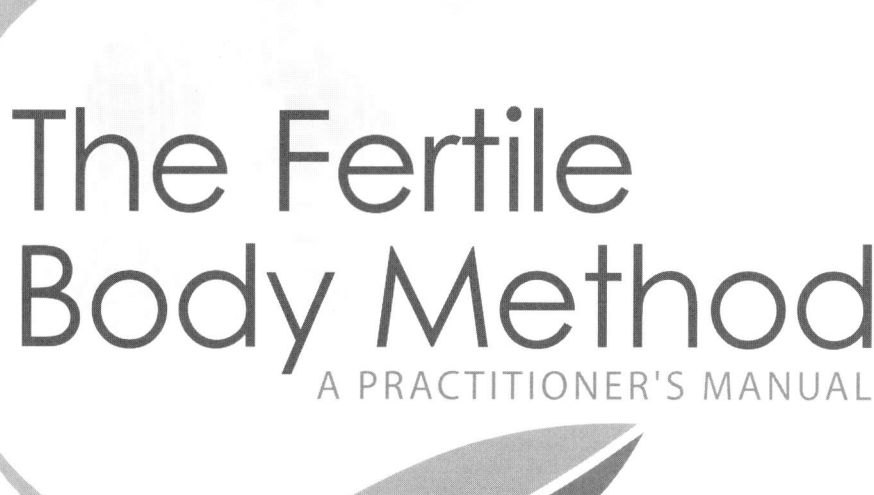

# The Fertile Body Method
## A PRACTITIONER'S MANUAL

The applications of hypnosis and other mind-body approaches for fertility

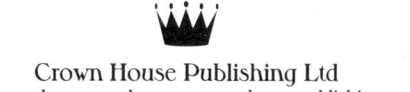

Crown House Publishing Ltd
www.crownhouse.co.uk   www.crownhousepublishing.com

First published by

Crown House Publishing Ltd
Crown Buildings, Bancyfelin, Carmarthen, Wales, SA33 5ND, UK
www.crownhouse.co.uk

and

Crown House Publishing Company LLC
6 Trowbridge Drive, Suite 5, Bethel, CT 06801-2858, USA
www.crownhousepublishing.com

© Sjanie Hugo 2009

The right of Sjanie Hugo to be identified as the author of this work has been asserted by her in accordance with the Copyright, Designs and Patents Act 1988.

All rights reserved. Apart from the handouts and worksheets provided on the CD accompanying this work and except as permitted under current legislation, no part of this work may be photocopied, stored in a retrieval system, published, performed in public, adapted, broadcast, transmitted, recorded or reproduced in any form or by any means, without the prior permission of the copyright owner.
Enquiries should be addressed to
Crown House Publishing Limited.

The *7:11 Breathing* script (Page 183) and *Rewind Technique* (Page 206) have been reproduced with kind permission of Joe Griffin and Ivan Tyrrell. *Resource Gathering* (Page 194) and *Anchor* (Page 216) have been reproduced with kind permission of Meta Publications. *Control Room* (Page 200), *Regressions – free floating* (Page 208), *Apposition of Opposites* (Page 218), *Free Floating pseudo-orientation in time* (Page 231) and *The Storm Cloud* (Page 235) have been reproduced with the kind permission of the London College of Clinical Hypnosis. *Somatic Bridge Regression* (Page 214) has been reproduced with the kind permission of Lynsi Eastburn. *Grief Ceremony* (Page 284) has been reproduced with kind permission of Niravi Payne. *Hypothalamus Meditation* (Page 244) has been reproduced with the kind permission of Llewellyn Publications (*The Mind-Body Fertility Connection: the True Pathway to Conception* by James Schwartz ©2008 Llewellyn Worldwide, Ltd. 2143 Wooddale Drive, Woodbury, MN 55125-2989. All rights reserved, used by permission and with the best wishes of the publisher). *Polarity Exercise* (Page 221) has been reproduced with the kind permission of Gosia Gorna. *Three Steps Forward* (Page 223) from *Fertile Heart ® Imagery* CD has been reproduced with the kind permission of Julia Indichova. *Bird Cage Release* (Page 246) and *Cellular Memory Recall* (Page 248) have been reproduced with kind permission of Julie Cleasby. Illustrations on pages 303 and 307 are used with kind permission and are from *The Merck Manual of Medical Information* - Second Home edition, edited by Robert S. Porter ©2007 by
Merck and Co.Inc., Whitehouse Staton NJ Available at www.merck.com/mmhe.

**British Library Cataloguing-in-Publication Data**
A catalogue entry for this book is available
from the British Library.

**ISBN 978-184590096-0**

**LCCN 2008936803**

Printed and bound in the UK by
*Cromwell Press Group, Trowbridge, Wiltshire*

# CONTENTS

**A Brief Summary** ...................................................................................................i
Foreword ..................................................................................................................iii

**Section A: Introduction** ......................................................................................1
   A mind-body approach to fertility ................................................................2
   An overview of the *Fertile Body Method* .....................................................3
   How the *Fertile Body Method* can help fertility problems ........................6
   The role of hypnosis in therapy ......................................................................8
   What is infertility? ...........................................................................................13

**Section B: The Stages Of Treatment** .............................................................23
   Stage 1: Outcome ............................................................................................25
      Set the goal ................................................................................................26
      Assess the information ............................................................................38
      Inform the client ........................................................................................49
   Stage 2: Balance ..............................................................................................55
      Factors affecting the fertile state ............................................................56
      Beliefs, emotions and the body ..............................................................59
      Approaches to create balance .................................................................62
   Stage 3: Resolve ..............................................................................................89
      The importance of resolution for fertility ............................................91
      Who is to blame? ......................................................................................94
      How to identify issues that may need to be resolved ........................95
      Some possible approaches for resolution ............................................96
      Some possible issues to resolve .............................................................98
      Some possible areas of inner conflict ....................................................98
      Unconscious blocks ..................................................................................99
      Age .............................................................................................................103
      Previous termination .............................................................................105
      Miscarriage ..............................................................................................108
      Stillbirth and neonatal death ...............................................................114
      Menstrual health ....................................................................................115
      Parenthood ..............................................................................................123
   Stage 4: Enhance ...........................................................................................125
      Visualisation approaches to enhance fertility ...................................126
      Considerations when working with visualisation approaches .......127
      The applications of visualisation approaches for fertility ...............129
      Visualisation scripts to enhance fertility ............................................132
      Working with physical problems to enhance fertility .....................133
   Stage 5: Prepare .............................................................................................137
      Preparation for pregnancy ...................................................................138
      Preparation for birth ..............................................................................143
      Preparation for parenthood .................................................................149
      Preparation for medical treatments ....................................................154

Stage 6: Support ..................................................................................157
　　　　Support to maintain change .........................................................158
　　　　How to maintain change ..............................................................159
　　　　The importance of emotional support ........................................162
　　　　Support during pregnancy ..........................................................163
　　　　Support after miscarriage and stillbirth ....................................164
　　　　IVF and other medical treatment failure ...................................165
　　　　Choosing not to become parents ................................................167
　　　　Looking at the options for parenthood .....................................171
　　　　Moving on ......................................................................................173

　　Working with men .................................................................................177

**Section C: Techniques, Scripts And Tools** ...........................................181
　　Techniques and scripts ..........................................................................181
　　Self-help tools .........................................................................................279

**Section D: Paths To Parenthood** ...........................................................295
　　Paths to parenthood ..............................................................................296
　　Things you may need to know about natural conception ................300
　　Assisted Reproductive Technology (ART) .........................................308

**Section E: Resources** ...............................................................................349
　　Recommended reading .........................................................................351
　　Useful websites ......................................................................................355
　　Further study and support ...................................................................359
　　Glossary of terms ...................................................................................361
　　Bibliography ...........................................................................................371
　　Index ........................................................................................................377
　　Acknowledgements ...............................................................................387
　　Data CD
　　　　Questionnaire – for men and woman
　　　　Scripts and techniques – for therapists to customise and print
　　　　Self-help tools – guide sheet handouts for clients
　　　　Fertility Awareness Education Programme – handout for clients
　　　　Finding meaning, purpose and direction – homework questions

## *A brief summary*

The *Fertile Body Method* combines hypnosis and other mind-body approaches to help identify and address the mental, emotional and physical factors which affect fertility and reduce the negative effects of infertility.

This book is a manual for health practitioners and contains the six stages of the '*Fertile Body Method*', which can be used to study, understand and work with all the different aspects of fertility problems. This manual includes a structured therapeutic framework as well as a step-by-step guide for treatment. It is packed with tips, suggestions, tools and techniques which will provide practitioners with practical ways of working with each stage of treatment. The lively case studies illustrate some of the ways that this therapeutic framework can be put into practice.

## *Who is this book for?*

This book is primarily aimed at hypnotherapists and mental health practitioners who work with, or are interested in working with hypnosis and mind-body approaches for fertility. It is also valuable for other health practitioners wanting to learn more about the mind-body relationship and how we can use the mind to enhance fertility. This book is suitable for those who are new to the field of fertility and mind-body medicine as well as more experienced practitioner's who are looking to add to their skills and knowledge.

Many of the approaches suggested in the book utilise a hypnotic state. If you are not a trained hypnotherapist I would recommend that you do not work with formal hypnosis. However, many of these techniques can be used successfully in a state of deep relaxation. All the techniques marked 'can be used without formal hypnosis' may be suitable for use by practitioners who are experienced with guided relaxation and guided visualisation approaches.

## How to use this manual

This book is divided into five sections as follows:

- **Section A** introduces hypnosis, mind-body medicine and explains fertility and infertility.

- **Section B** contains the six stages of the *Fertile Body Method*.

- **Section C** includes detailed descriptions of all the techniques, scripts and self-help tools referred to within the book.

- **Section D** outlines the different paths to parenthood and looks specifically at working with natural conception and assisted conception.

- **Section E** includes useful resources and a CD. The CD contains many practical resources such as scripts, questionnaires and homework sheets that can be printed out for your sessions or to be given as handouts to your clients.

I recommend that you read all the chapters before using the techniques and methods, in order to make a positive difference to your patient's health and fertility.

## About the author

Sjanie Hugo is a clinical hypnotherapist specialising in fertility and related issues. She works in a busy central London practice and also works as part of a team at an integrated fertility clinic in London. She has lectured internationally for The London College of Clinical Hypnosis (LCCH).

Sjanie developed the *Fertile Body Method* and runs training courses throughout the UK and abroad where she teaches this approach to other practitioners. Sjanie also co-runs the 'Fertile Being' group workshops using the concepts outlined in the *Fertile Body Method* to directly work with and empower couples who want to have children.

Sjanie is particularly interested in the healing affects of movement and dance and is undergoing personal study with the School of Movement Medicine.

## *Foreword*

I remember being 14 years old, sitting in a biology class taught by my teacher Mrs Zondagh. We had spent the year studying different species and looking at how they reproduce. We'd covered everything from the earthworm to large mammals. And finally we were going to be looking at human reproduction. It was a very exciting day for most of us because at last we were going to be able to talk about sex. As a teenager I was rather mischievous and enjoyed finding ways to cause commotion at this 'proper' girls' high school. I spent the morning planning what questions I would ask during the lesson. My aim was to try to say the rudest thing possible in a way that would come across as a genuine interest to learn, without getting reprimanded or punished.

While these questions kept me very amused throughout the class, there was something Mrs Zondagh said that day that really stuck in my mind. With a serious look on her face she said, 'Your whole purpose is to reproduce. You were born to reproduce. It is all about finding the right boy, and making babies with him.' I was horrified by this statement, thinking that there really MUST be more to life than that. Now, looking back, I get her point. Every living organism is designed to reproduce. Without reproduction the species could die. Survival of our species is a deep innate drive. It certainly is one of our primary urges. Of course, as conscious beings we are able to choose not to follow that urge. And fortunately there are many different ways that we can find purpose and meaning in our lives. But because this desire to reproduce is so ingrained in us, both instinctively and culturally, it is understandable why infertility can be the source of so much pain and sadness.

Approximately one in six couples in the United Kingdom is having problems conceiving and many of them are actively seeking help. I have written this book so that other practitioners working with fertility problems can have access to information that I believe is invaluable when working with these clients.

The approaches I present in this book combine many different schools of thought, and have been influenced by a variety of people. My interest in science, along with my personal experiences with acupuncture, trance, healing and dance have strongly influenced my life and the way in which I work. All of the things that I have learnt and experienced and found to be helpful have been woven together to create the *Fertile Body Method*.

Essentially I believe that there are many possible factors that affect fertility. The role of the mind and the emotions in fertility is a vital one that is often overlooked. I am not suggesting that the sole reason for fertility problems is 'in the mind' or that couples must have done something 'wrong' to have found themselves having difficulty conceiving. Rather I am suggesting that a truly integrated approach is far more likely to give people the best possible chance of having children.

The approaches in this book are aimed at helping couples to deal with the effects of fertility problems and make changes that can help to positively impact on their fertility. Although I obviously can't guarantee that the *Fertile Body Method* will result in the client having a baby, I do know that it will make the process easier and help them to handle the outcome better, irrespective of what that might be. Through the therapeutic process it is often possible for people to experience deep healing and positive inner changes irrespective of whether they have children or not.

I feel it is worth mentioning that this book is a collection of ideas and suggestions and offers *a way* of approaching fertility problems. It isn't conclusive, nor is it complete, and it certainly does not answer all the questions.

I realise that irrespective of your background and experience, you will have your own ideas and opinions. Perhaps you will strongly disagree with some of the things I say, or perhaps you will find that what I am saying resonates with what you already know. I would love to hear your ideas and comments so please feel free to contact me directly to share your knowledge and experience. In a future updated version of this book I hope to include many more contributions from other therapists.

## Author's note

The case studies throughout the book are based on clients with whom I have worked. To protect their anonymity, and for teaching purposes, I have in some cases changed some of the details of the case.

Although fertility problems affect both men and women, the majority of the clients I see for therapy are women. For ease of reading I refer to 'woman' and 'her' rather than 'woman/man' and 'her/him', but much of this information is equally valid and useful for working with both sexes. There are some issues which specifically affect men and are addressed in *Working with men* in Section B.

## Section A: Introduction

This section introduces the *Fertile Body Method* and explains some of the concepts behind this mind-body approach to fertility. Along with a summary of how the *Fertile Body Method* can help those with fertility problems, I have included a description of hypnosis and some ideas on how it works and how it can be used therapeutically for those who are not familiar with hypnotherapy.

For those who are new to the field of fertility I have included some information about infertility, the scale of the problem, possible causes, medical tests and the effects of infertility on people's lives. Information about the male and female reproductive system and the physiology of conception can be found in *Section D: Paths to Parenthood* (Page 295).

**This section contains:**
- A mind-body approach to fertility ...........................................2
- An overview of the *Fertile Body Method* .........................................3
- How the *Fertile Body Method* can help fertility problems ....................6
- The role of hypnosis in therapy ...............................................8
- What is infertility? ...............................................................13

## *A mind-body approach to fertility*

> *Mind-body medicine is any method in which we use our minds to change our behaviours or physiology in order to promote health or recover from illness.*
> Alice Domar (Domar, 2002, p. 41)

Viewing health as more than a physical issue is certainly not a new concept. From my own personal experience it is easy to recognise that health is experienced as mental, emotional, spiritual and physical wellbeing. Many cultures throughout the world use a medical model that fully acknowledges the inter-connectedness between these different aspects of our being.

After René Descartes proposed that the mind and body operate separately with no interconnectedness, the body began to be seen as a machine that could be mechanically fixed. This attitude towards the body has dominated much of Western medicine and given rise to mechanistic approaches to fertility, such as IVF. While these kinds of treatments can be a wonderful way to address biological problems affecting fertility, they have, in some ways, continued to propagate the myth that the body, and indeed fertility, are mechanical.

Mind-body medicine is an approach to health that recognises the effect that our mind has on our body, and vice versa. This model views the various aspects of ourselves and the different systems of our body, as a part of the greater whole. This holistic approach acknowledges the effect that one part, or one system, will have on another. It recognises that a human being is a dynamic living organism that strives to maintain balance and wellbeing through obtaining the right physical and emotional nourishment from its environment and incorporating it correctly into its system.

Problems with conception and pregnancy can occur when our basic physical and emotional needs are not being met and the mind and/or body have temporarily lost their natural state of balance and harmony. Imbalance may be caused by external environmental factors, unhealthy internal processes or the inability to get one's basic physical and emotional needs met in a healthy way.

> *It is almost always a mistake to look for a single cause to a problem or an imbalance or an illness. Not only is it usually wrong to think of "one illness one cause", but it is also invariably insufficient to use one therapy or one health maintenance plan. Carefully co-ordinated combinations [of treatment] are key. Once you learn how to use combinations the effects can be magnificent.*
> Dr Richard G. Petty, (Petty, 2007)

## *An overview of the* Fertile Body Method

The *Fertile Body Method* is a mind-body approach to fertility problems that is based on a holistic health model. It acknowledges the importance of working together with other specialists to create well co-ordinated combinations of treatments.

The *Fertile Body Method* has grown out of my experience of working with many couples who have had difficulty conceiving. My particular 'style' of therapy combines a variety of psychotherapeutic approaches with other forms of healing that I have learnt and/or benefitted from personally. In order to share what I know, and make this information useful for other therapists, I have developed a therapeutic framework consisting of six stages of treatment that will allow each therapist to apply their own unique style and experience.

The structure is designed to be safe, flexible and effective and, as such, should give therapists a solid foundation on which to build. I believe that plans and structures are a valuable part of any creative process and should always be used as a way to enhance what you do. If a plan or structure becomes limiting, it may indicate the need for a new plan. I mention this because I recognise that the therapeutic process is a creative one, which is alive and changing in the moment. Having the safety of a structure can help you to really be present to the process and allow creative and intuitive responses to arise.

I hope that the *Fertile Body Method* provides you with a framework that will guide you but still allow you to respond creatively and intuitively to your clients.

The Fertile Body Method

## *Stages of treatment*

The therapeutic framework for the *Fertile Body Method* comprises six key stages:

1. *Outcome*
   The first stage is to determine the desired outcome for the hypnotherapy treatment. This includes setting the goal, gathering information, and determining the best possible course for treatment.

2. *Balance*
   The second stage of treatment addresses the client's current mental, emotional and physical state by restoring balance to internal and external factors that may be affecting overall wellbeing. This may include addressing negative self-talk, stress levels, diet, lifestyle and other environmental factors. The main aims of this stage are to stabilise the client, build ego strength, develop their inner resources and increase feelings of wellbeing.

3. *Resolve*
   Once greater psychological and emotional wellbeing has been established, the third treatment stage addresses any unresolved issues that may be preventing the couple from becoming parents. Important issues may include addressing fears, resolving past traumas, or dealing with sexual or relationship issues. During this stage of treatment you may work with issues such as previous terminations, miscarriages and stillbirths that have not been fully processed and integrated.

4. *Enhance*
   The fourth stage of treatment works specifically with the conscious and unconscious mind to enhance fertility. This is predominantly achieved through visualisation, guided imagery and *Mental Rehearsal*.

5. *Prepare*
   The fifth stage is focused on preparation. This preparation could be for pregnancy, birth or parenthood. It also includes mental, emotional and physical preparation for any medical treatments such as IVF.

6. *Support*
   The sixth stage of the treatment aims to support the client and help maintain the changes that they have made. This could be working with the client if conception does not occur; the pregnancy results in

> miscarriage; IVF fails or a healthy pregnancy ensues. Irrespective of the outcome of treatment, this final stage offers support and guidance for the transition. During this stage you may help the couple to make difficult decisions about their path to parenthood or support them in coming to terms with not having children.

*Stage 1: Outcome* and *Stage 2: Balance* form the essential foundations for treatment and, I believe, they should always be included in the treatment plan. The remaining stages do not need to be followed in sequence, and it may be appropriate to omit one or more stages of treatment. The sequence and the stages you choose to work with will be determined by the individual client and their goal for therapy.

I would however like to emphasise the importance of achieving an overall state of balance before proceeding with any other stages of treatment. Firstly, I believe that this is fundamental for fertility; and secondly, achieving balance and increased wellbeing will help to make available the resources needed to address the more challenging issues in *Stage 3: Resolve*.

While I present this Method in a very structured and linear way, the reality of how I work can sometimes be very different to this. The essential parts of this framework that I always bear in mind are: establishing the goal/outcome; building inner resources and creating stability before resolving any relevant issues. I believe that these components are what make the approach safe and effective.

## *How the* **Fertile Body Method** *can help fertility problems*

In summary, the *Fertile Body Method* can be used to help increase fertility and to address the negative effects of infertility.

> ### *It helps increase fertility by:*
>
> - Reducing stress and increasing feelings of calm and relaxation.
>
> - Restoring physical, mental and emotional balance and wellbeing
>   - Balance can be restored through relaxation, positive cognitive changes, visualisation and changes to diet, exercise and lifestyle.
>   - Overall wellbeing can be restored by ensuring that the client's physical and emotional needs are being met (Griffin and Tyrrell, 2004b).
>
> - Identifying and resolving issues that may be preventing conception (unconscious or conscious resistance). The following are examples of issues that may prevent conception:
>   - Fears about pregnancy, birth, parenthood
>   - Fears about ability to cope
>   - Concerns about work vs family
>   - Concerns about relationship
>   - Unresolved trauma
>   - Previous miscarriage, stillbirth or birth trauma
>   - Terminations
>   - Unresolved grief
>   - Unresolved issues from childhood
>   - Issues with own femininity/masculinity.
>
> - Preparing the couple for conception by helping them:
>   - To make the necessary changes to their lifestyle, diet, smoking, alcohol intake and exercise habits
>   - To feel confident and ready for parenthood
>   - To improve intimacy and their sexual relationship (for natural conception)
>   - To restore menstrual health, or sperm mobility and count
>   - To prepare for IVF or other fertility treatment.

- Providing support
  - Teaching self-help tools that continue to enhance fertility.
  - Support to maintain the changes they have made.
  - Supporting the couple if they do conceive in order to help carry the baby to full term.
  - Supporting them to make decisions about fertility treatments and other options for parenthood.

## *Address and reduce the effects of infertility*

People who have problems conceiving may experience a reduced sense of mental, emotional and physical wellbeing that leaves them feeling stressed, frustrated, angry, jealous, guilty, hopeless, anxious or depressed. It can affect their work, friendships, family and relationships. The negative effects of infertility can be reduced by:

- Restoring self-esteem and self-worth
- Working through emotions such as anger, jealousy, guilt, stress, anxiety and depression
- Building coping skills and developing inner resources
- Ensuring their physical and emotional needs are being met
- Resolving relationship problems (partner, family and friends)
- Increasing sexual intimacy and affection
- Restoring trust in one's body
- Reducing the negative effects of fertility treatment medication
- Restoring the body to good health after medical treatments
- Providing emotional support and an opportunity to talk openly
- Working through unresolved grief
- Coming to terms with infertility.

## The role of hypnosis in therapy

Hypnosis is a trance state induced through focusing attention on any current internal or external sensory experience; hypnotherapy is the art of utilising this state of absorption to facilitate inner change.

Hypnosis is potentially a very powerful and effective therapeutic tool and is used in many of the techniques and approaches suggested in the *Fertile Body Method*. I have included some information about hypnosis and its applications for those who are unfamiliar with hypnotherapy. While some of the techniques utilising formal hypnosis do require training in hypnotherapy, many others can be effectively used without formal hypnosis or by guiding the client into a state of deep relaxation.

### Inducing a hypnotic state

> *There are many ways of inducing a trance, you ask the patient to primarily give their attention to one particular idea. You get them to centre their attention on their own experiential learning ... to direct their attention to processes which are taking place within them. Thus you can induce a trance by directing a patient's attention to experiences, memories, ideas, and concepts that belong to them. All you do is direct their attention to those processes within themselves.*
> 
> Milton Erickson, M.D.

Trance states can be accessed in a variety of ways, many of which occur spontaneously. Hypnotic trance is a normal, natural state that we move into and out of many times in our daily life.

High emotional arousal induces a natural trance state because our attention becomes focused on the thing that has aroused us, giving us a singular perspective. The brain's rational function (originating in the neocortex) becomes less active, giving rise to more spontaneous, instinctive responses.

A trance state can also occur when we voluntarily choose to focus our attention on something that interests us. Any activity that absorbs our attention will induce a trance state, whether it is reading, watching TV, making love or dancing.

> *[The hypnotic state] is in evidence in everyday life whenever attention is fixated with a question or an experience of the amazing, the unusual, or anything that holds a person's interest. At such moments people experience the common everyday trance; they tend to gaze off to the right or left, depending upon which cerebral*

*hemisphere is most dominant (Baleen, 1969) and get that far away or blank look. Their eyes may actually close, their bodies tend to become immobile (a form of catalepsy), certain reflexes (e.g., swallowing, respiration, etc.) may be suppressed, and they seem momentarily oblivious to their surroundings until they have completed their inner search on the unconscious level for the new idea, response, or frames of reference that will restabilise their general reality orientation. We hypothesize that in everyday life consciousness is in a continual state of flux between the general reality orientation and the momentary microdynamics of trance.*

(Erickson and Rossi, 1976)

As well as trance arising spontaneously and voluntarily, a trance state can be induced when somebody else focuses our attention. This capacity stems from a primary survival need for us to be able to learn from others, be part of groups and absorb cultural norms. When our attention is guided by another in a compelling way we are likely to accept their suggestions (Griffin and Tyrrell, 2004b, p. 62). This gives us the capacity to learn things from others as well as from our own experience.

People are often guided into a state of hypnosis as they listen to words that help them focus their attention on the feelings of deepening relaxation. This helps to induce a pleasurable and comfortable therapeutic trance state that has the added benefit of relaxation.

When we enter a state of hypnosis by directing our attention towards increasing comfort, the parasympathetic nervous system is activated, giving rise to what is known as the relaxation response. When the relaxation response is activated we enter a state of deep physical relaxation. This response works in opposition to the 'fight or flight response' and counteracts the body's physical and emotional response to stress, allowing it to return to a calm balanced state. While in this state there is a measurable decrease in heart rate, blood pressure, breathing rate, stress hormone levels and muscle tension and people experience a wonderful feeling of relaxation.

## *What does hypnosis feel like?*

*Hypnosis is a peaceful, creative and productive state of inner absorption. It is a natural learning state that occurs from within. Hypnosis is a natural human ability, and a powerful tool for change.*

Stephen Gilligan (Gilligan, 1997)

Hypnosis can be experienced to varying depths and is experienced differently from person to person. While in a state of hypnosis we can be aware of what is going on around us, although we are likely to become so absorbed in our own inner experience that we choose to pay little attention to unnecessary distractions.

While in a hypnotic state we can hear everything that is being said, but afterwards we may not necessarily remember everything that was said. This kind of amnesia occurs spontaneously, in the same way that we only selectively remember events and conversations from our daily life. We choose to remember only the things that are important for us to remember consciously.

The hypnotic state is often characterised by a distorted experience of time. We experience perceived time as substantially longer or shorter than actual time. Most commonly we experience a long time spent in trance as having passed by very quickly. Similarly when we are enjoying an experience, time just seems to fly by.

Other common phenomena and experiences of hypnosis include analgesia (partial loss of sensation), anaesthesia (total loss of sensation), catalepsy (automatic contraction and apparent paralysis of muscles) and dissociation (feeling separated from one's immediate ordinary sensory experience and environment).

While in this state we may be able to recall things more vividly and easily and are more likely to remember events with all our senses. This sometimes gives us the feeling that we are reliving the event as if we were experiencing it right now. For this reason, imagined events can feel quite 'real'.

In many respects, being in a state of hypnosis is a very ordinary and extraordinary experience, one which is likely to feel familiar or similar to what we have experienced before. People who have experienced guided visualisation or other meditative states describe it as being similar to hypnosis in many ways. Ultimately, the only true way to know what hypnosis feels like is to experience it. And the more often we experience the trance state, the deeper it is likely to become.

## *The conscious and the unconscious mind*

The conscious and the unconscious are the terms used to describe the different aspects of our mind.

The conscious mind is the active mind that can think different thoughts. It is the mind that holds our current and immediate experience and awareness. This awareness can include thoughts, feelings and sensory experiences. The unconscious mind is the storehouse of all our past, present and future experiences of which we are presently unaware. The unconscious also holds our automatic behaviours as a set of stimulus-response 'programmes', if you like, which have been derived from our instincts and learned experiences. The unconscious mind is strictly habitual and will automatically respond to life's signals over and over again.

Milton Erickson believed that the innate intelligence that keeps our heart beating, our body breathing and all other automated functions in place resides in the unconscious mind.

In terms of neurological processing abilities, the unconscious mind is a million times more powerful than the conscious mind. If the desires of the conscious mind conflict with the unconscious, the unconscious mind will dominate (Lipton, 2005, p. 128).

Hypnosis is an effective tool for creating change on an unconscious level, using visualisations, suggestions and other cognitive, behavioural and analytical tools.

## *The therapeutic applications of hypnosis*

The therapeutic applications of hypnosis are only limited by our imagination. It is a tool that can be used in a variety of ways to treat a wide range of issues. This section describes some of the general applications of hypnosis.

- The state of hypnosis can itself be therapeutic. When we enter a state of hypnosis by directing our attention towards increasing comfort, the parasympathetic nervous system is activated, giving rise to the relaxation response. This response works in opposition to the fight or flight response and counteracts the body's physical and emotional response to stress, allowing it to return to a calm balanced state. Simply being in the state of hypnosis will create physiological changes that reduce stress and its negative effects on health and wellbeing.

- Another added benefit of hypnotic relaxation, is that it reduces emotional arousal such as anger or fear. During a state of high emotional arousal the brain's cortical functions become limited and we lose our ability to reason. Relaxation reduces the arousal giving us access to our higher rational abilities. It is for this reason that we are more likely to gain perspective and reach new insight and understanding while in a hypnotic state.

- The hypnotic state allows us to communicate with or access our unconscious mind so that we can recall past experiences, access our inner wisdom and tap into our personal resources. This hypnotic ability means that we can draw on each client's unique history to help them receive more of what it is they need in current and future situations. For example, to help them build confidence or increase motivation.

- Since our higher cortical functions are activated and our unconscious resources are more readily available to us in a state of hypnosis, we are more easily able to find solutions and resolve problems.

- All of our habitual and automatic behaviours are stored in the unconscious. Hypnotherapy can be used to decondition habits and to create new automatic behaviours and responses. For example, this could be particularly useful to reduce the anxiety response in the case of a phobia.

- The beliefs we hold are like the device that helps run the 'programmes' containing our automatic responses. By integrating successful cognitive therapy approaches, we can use hypnotherapy to challenge unhealthy beliefs and find new beliefs that will create healthier automatic responses to situations and events.

- During hypnosis our imagination and creative abilities are enhanced. We can use this vivid imagination to see ourselves thinking, feeling and behaving in the way we would like to in future situations. Using hypnosis for positive *Mental Rehearsal* can create a healthy mental and physiological response when that situation is encountered again in real life. This is particularly useful for future situations that previously provoked anxiety, fear, dread or concern. *Positive Mental Rehearsal* will improve our future responses as well as reduce the anxiety caused when we think about the event.

- Past disturbing or traumatic events that continue to carry an emotional charge for us can be resolved using hypnotherapy. These experiences can be integrated so that the necessary learning remains, but the emotional and energetic arousal is reduced. Resolving and integrating these past experiences allows us to live without the negative impact of that event affecting our present life.

- In a state of hypnosis, our inner senses become heightened and allow us to become more sensitive to our own subtle experiences. We can use this sensitivity to become more aware of our physical body and its messages to us. We know that there are many ways in which we can use the mind to create changes in the body. Guided visualisation is a well-known approach which uses the mind, and specifically the imagination, as a means of creating physical change. And so, in the above-mentioned ways, we can use hypnosis to alleviate any physical conditions, illness or pain.

- One of the great strengths of hypnotherapy is that hypnosis is a tool that can be learnt. Once the client has learnt to induce a state of hypnosis on their own, they can use this tool to benefit themselves on an ongoing basis. They can learn a variety of ways in which they can use hypnosis to reinforce changes and continue to facilitate new and positive learning.

## *What is infertility?*

If you are intending to work with clients who have fertility problems, they will generally expect you to have a reasonable knowledge of infertility, the possible causes, medical tests and other factors that can affect it. Many of those who have been struggling to conceive for some time will be exceptionally clued up about the medical facts. In order to maintain good rapport and work effectively, I would recommend gaining a good understanding of infertility and the relevant medical terminology.

When I first began working in this field I was amazed at how much my clients knew about their medical diagnosis and treatment. Interestingly, many of them were less knowledgeable about the biological facts of natural conception. I have found that as my fertility knowledge has grown, I have been able to build greater trust and rapport.

To find out more about the anatomy and physiology of conception please refer to *Things you may need to know about natural conception* in Section D (Page 300). For more in-depth information about infertility and related problems, please refer to the recommended reading list in Section E (Page 351).

## Infertility defined

Infertility is defined as the *'diminished ability or the inability to conceive and have offspring. Infertility is also defined in specific terms as the failure to conceive after a year of regular intercourse without contraception.'* (MedicineNet.com, 2003)

- Typically the term *infertility* is used to describe the inability to conceive.

- *Subfertility* is a term that is used in the medical field and indicates that there are problems that make conception difficult if not highly unlikely without medical help. This term is also used if you can get pregnant but keep having miscarriages.

- *Primary infertility* is used to describe a couple that has never been able to conceive after at least one year of unprotected intercourse.

- *Secondary infertility* describes couples who, after having had one or more babies, can't conceive or who have had one or more miscarriages or stillbirths. Secondary infertility is more common than primary infertility.

Approximately 32% of fertility problems are due to female factors, 32% due to male factors, 11% combined male and female factors and 24% of cases have no obvious cause associated with them, leading to a diagnosis of unexplained infertility. (Human Fertilisation and Embryology Authority (HFEA), 2008).

The diagnosis of *unexplained infertility* is made after one year of unprotected sex and when tests have been carried out on both partners and no biological problems have been found.

Unexplained infertility could be explained in some of the following ways:

- There is a biological or environmental factor that medics are not yet aware of that is causing the infertility.

- The couple have just been 'unlucky'.

- They are not having sex during the woman's fertile time.

- Psychological and emotional factors are causing fertility problems.

## The scale of fertility problems

It is estimated that one in six UK couples have difficulty conceiving – about 3.5 million people. Though the majority of these will become pregnant naturally given time, a significant minority will not (HFEA, 2008).

Of 100 couples trying to conceive naturally:

- After one month, 20% will have conceived
- After six months, 70% will have conceived
- After a year, 85% will have conceived
- After 18 months, 90% will have conceived
- After two years, 95% will have conceived.

(These statistics are published in conjunction with the *HFEA Guide to Infertility* treatment and success data based on treatment carried out in 2005.)

## The impact of infertility

Every person is affected differently by infertility, depending upon the beliefs they hold, their current circumstances and the emotional, physical and social resources they have available to them. Infertility can affect every aspect of your client's life, from their relationship with their partner, family and friends to their career.

The desire to have children is an innate biological drive and is reinforced through cultural conditioning. Having difficulties conceiving or carrying a baby to full term can affect people on a very primal level. Being told that you are 'infertile' will most certainly affect the way your client feels about themselves and may make them question their value and worth.

The pressures of trying to conceive may affect their relationship emotionally and sexually. In an attempt to do everything they can to conceive, they will make many sacrifices and changes to their lifestyle. Often this includes doing less of the things they used to enjoy, which they think may be bad for their fertility. If they find themselves becoming upset easily around friends who are pregnant or have babies, they may choose to avoid seeing them, so often their social network becomes smaller and smaller at a time when they most need the support of friends. In cases where family members are insensitive, or are adding to the pressure of trying to conceive, couples may choose to see them less.

Medical treatments are very time consuming and often require your clients to be available often at short notice. This can create stress and difficulties at work, especially if they have chosen not to tell their employer about what they are going through. Tests and medical treatments can also be a financial burden. Often couples have to borrow huge sums of money to pay for treatment and the financial pressure can lead to further stress. Medical interventions will have a physical effect on their bodies and may disrupt their overall health.

There are constant reminders everywhere about what it is they want and can't have. For women there is also the monthly reminder at the time of menstruation that she has not conceived. The ongoing struggle can leave your client feeling out of control and hopeless. Stress and depression can continue to build as beliefs about never having children grow. For many, infertility is an emotional roller-coaster of hope and disappointment that seems never-ending.

## *The causes of infertility*

A wide variety of factors affect fertility, and there are many potential causes of infertility. These range from physical and chemical factors to subtle energy, emotional and psychological factors. In Section B, *Stage 2: Balance* we will look at the psychological and emotional factors in more detail. For more information about the male and female reproductive system please refer to Section D.

*Some common physical causes for women include:*

- Abnormal ovulation: occurs when the egg-production cycle is not functioning normally due to hormonal deficiencies or imbalances. Ovulation and the hormonal changes that follow are responsible for maintaining a normal menstrual cycle. Irregular periods strongly suggest that an egg is not being released each month. It is also possible that ovulation may not be occurring (anovulation) even when the cycle appears normal. Anovulation may be the result of an overactive pituitary gland, leading to high levels of the hormone prolactin. Where the ovary has exhausted its egg supply and premature ovarian failure is the diagnosis, the only treatment is IVF with donor eggs.

- Polycystic Ovarian Syndrome (PCOS): PCOS is now recognised as one of the most common causes of ovulation failure. In polycystic ovarian syndrome, many follicles are produced but often none develop enough to release an egg, meaning that ovulation does not take place. Hormone production is also often unbalanced, particularly with raised levels of androgens such as testosterone.

- Damaged Fallopian tubes: blockage or scarring of the tubes can prevent the egg and sperm from uniting or may prevent the united egg and sperm from descending to the uterus for maturation (resulting in an ectopic pregnancy). The most common cause of blocked tubes is infection, most commonly with chlamydia. About 70% of women who have blocked tubes have had chlamydia, although half the time it will have been silent and they will not have even been aware of it. Where the tubes look otherwise normal and the blockage is close to the uterus, or where scar tissue adhesions are causing a distinct blockage, surgical correction is sometimes possible.

- Pelvic inflammatory disease (PID): this umbrella term refers to an inflammation of any of the pelvic organs, including the reproductive organs, which can impede their ability to facilitate conception or support a pregnancy.

- Endometriosis: occurs when the uterine lining (or endometrium) grows outside the uterus, resulting in excess bleeding, blockage, or scarring in the surrounding reproductive structures, which can interfere with conception or pregnancy. Although extensive endometriosis involving the Fallopian tubes and the ovaries are clearly likely to interfere with ovulation and egg transport, it is less clear how mild to moderate endometriosis exerts an effect on fertility. Surgical interventions to remove endometriosis are done by either cutting it out or burning it away with diathermy or laser, breaking down any associated adhesions and leaving as much normal ovarian tissue as possible. Mild to moderate endometriosis can usually be managed laparoscopically, but more severe cases require open surgery.

- Hostile cervical mucus: the cervical mucus is a jelly-like substance produced by minute glands in the cervical canal. It changes in consistency and composition with the menstrual cycle. Just before ovulation and under the effect of the hormone oestrogen it becomes very watery and copious to allow the sperm to swim through it. Hostile cervical mucus is a term that describes mucus that impedes the natural progression of the sperm within the cervical canal. The mucus may be too acidic or too sticky and thick, thereby preventing the sperm from flowing freely throughout the cervix. This can be caused by a number of factors and some examples may include poor oestrogen stimulation or perhaps an infection which prevents the cervical glands from operating properly.

- Incidental causes: these causes include damage inflicted on any part of the reproductive system by abdominal disease (such as Crohn's disease), surgery, therapy (such as chemotherapy), tumour (such as fibroid tumour), physical trauma, or drug exposure.

*Some common physical causes for infertility in men include:*

- Idiopathic low sperm count (unknown cause of a reduced sperm count): a commonly observed fertility abnormality in the male probably caused by an unknown intra-uterine factor that adversely affected the development of the testes during the male's embryonic life. Unfortunately, if bacterial cultures are negative, and the hormones are normal, and there is no varicocele (abnormal enlargement of the vein), there is currently no available treatment.

- Low sperm count: low sperm count (oligospermia) is a potential contributing factor to infertility. A normal sperm count is 20 million or more sperm per millilitre of semen. While sperm count is important for fertility, it is equally important that a good number of those sperm should have a normal shape (morphology) and show normal forward movement (motility).

- Poor sperm morphology: sperm morphology is routinely evaluated as part of a standard semen analysis. Morphology indicates the percentage of sperm that appear normal when semen is viewed under a microscope. Morphological defects may impair the ability of the sperm to reach and fertilise the egg.

- Dilated veins around the testicles: this condition, known as varicocele, increases the temperature in the scrotum, which can result in fewer sperm as well as malformed or malfunctioning sperm (what is commonly known as 'poor swimmers').

- Damaged sperm ducts: blockage or scarring in the sperm ducts (or vas deferens) prevents the sperm from reaching the seminal fluid.

- Hormone deficiency: an insufficient or too-erratic release of the hormones (including testosterone, LH and FSH) that stimulate sperm production.

- Retrograde ejaculation: this occurs when impairment of the muscles or nerves of the bladder neck prohibit it from closing during ejaculation, allowing semen to flow backwards into the bladder. It may result from bladder surgery, a developmental defect in the urethra or bladder, or disease that affects the nervous system, including diabetes. Signs of this condition may be diminished or 'dry' ejaculation and cloudy urine after ejaculation.

- Impotence: an inability to ejaculate inside the vagina due to physiological factors (such as hardening of the arteries, high blood pressure, diabetes, kidney disease, erectile dysfunction), environmental factors (such as substance abuse or certain medication regimens), or psychological factors (such as performance anxiety or premature ejaculation).

- Sperm antibodies: in rare cases (for example, among a small fraction of men who have undergone vasectomy reversals), the immune system develops antibodies to the sperm that kills the sperm as soon as it's produced.

- Incidental causes: this includes any damage caused by abdominal disease, surgery, therapy (such as chemotherapy), tumour, drug exposure, or physical trauma.

*Other external factors affecting fertility include:*

- Weight: being overweight or underweight.

- Nutrition: nutrient and mineral deficiency.

- General health: including the negative effects of hormone therapies like the contraceptive pill. There are also some illnesses which are known to affect fertility such as Crohn's disease.

- Age: a woman's fertility peaks in her 20s. As she gets older, and her health decreases, her fertility is likely to decrease, too. After the menopause a woman is no longer fertile.

- Toxins: environmental toxins as well as toxins in the body can have a negative effect on the hormonal system and affect fertility.

- Drug and alcohol use.

- Tobacco use.

- Physical exercise: in excess or a lack thereof.

## *Medical tests for infertility*

When a couple has been having regular unprotected sex for more than one year (for under 35) or six months (over 35), their GP is likely to refer them to a specialist to undergo a variety of tests to determine if there are any physical problems that may be affecting their fertility.

*Tests for women may include:*

- Measuring basal body temperature: taking the woman's temperature each morning before rising in an attempt to note the 0.4 to 1.0 degree Fahrenheit temperature increase associated with ovulation.

- Monitoring cervical mucus changes throughout the menstrual cycle to note the wet, stretchy, slippery mucus associated with the ovulatory phase.

- Blood test to check ovulation by measuring serum progesterone seven days before an expected period.

- Measuring the amount of luteinising hormone in urine with home-use kits to predict ovulation and assist with timing of intercourse. For more detailed information on the female reproductive system refer to Section D (Page 295) and the Fertility Awareness Education programme on the accompanying CD.

- Progestin challenge when the woman has sporadic or absent ovulation. Progestin is a synthetic pill form of the hormone progesterone which is taken by mouth once a day for five or more days to see if it triggers menstruation. When the progestin is stopped, bleeding ensues if oestrogen is present. If bleeding does not occur, then insufficient oestrogen is the probable cause of menstrual irregularity/absence.

- Postcoital testing (PCT) to evaluate sperm-cervical mucus interaction through the analysis of cervical mucus collected two to eight hours after the couple has had intercourse.

- Hysteroscopy: an operation to inspect the inside of the uterus, using a small telescope, to detect fibroid tumours, polyps, scarring and malignancies.

- Hysterosalpingography (HSG): an X-ray procedure done with contrast dye that looks at the route of sperm from the cervix through the uterus and Fallopian tubes. The HSG can help diagnose Fallopian tube blockages and defects of the uterus.

- Sono-hysterogram (SHG): a transvaginal (through the vagina) ultrasound using sound waves to determine if the uterus is normal in size and shape and is also used to diagnose Fallopian tube blockages.

- Laparoscopy to allow direct visualisation of the pelvic cavity to detect endometriosis, scarring and other abnormalities.

- Transvaginal (pelvic) ultrasound exam to determine whether the follicles in the ovaries are working normally. This is often performed 15 days before a woman's expected menstrual period.

- Endometrial biopsy: a biopsy of the uterine lining (endometrium) to see if it's normal.

*Tests for men may include:*

- Semen analysis: the specimen is collected after two to three days of complete abstinence to determine:
    - Motility: the sperm's swimming ability
    - Morphology: the shape of the sperm
    - Count/concentration: the number of individual sperm
    - Vitality: the capacity of the sperm to live.

- Ultrasound: to detect a blockage in the male ducts. A vasography (testicular biopsy) is a procedure that is used if the ultrasound is uncertain.

- Testicular biopsy: to determine if the testicles are producing sperm. This test is only done if no sperm is seen in the ejaculate and both ductal obstruction and retrograde ejaculation (condition in which semen is ejaculated into the bladder instead of exiting the body through the penis) are ruled out.

*Tests for men and women include:*

- Immunobead test (IBT): to check for the presence of antisperm antibodies. To detect antibodies, blood is drawn from the woman, incubated with a sperm sample and examined under a microscope in the laboratory.

## Section B: The Stages of Treatment

Section B contains all six stages of the *Fertile Body Method*. Each stage includes an in-depth description, with possible areas to address, useful techniques, therapeutic approaches and case study examples. A description of the scripts, techniques and self-help tools which are referred to throughout the book in italics can be found in Section C (Page 181). At the end of this section I have included information about working with men which addresses some of the fertility-related issues which affect them.

**This section contains:**
- Stage 1: Outcome .................................................................................................25
    - Set the goal ....................................................................................................26
    - Assess the information .................................................................................38
    - Inform the client ...........................................................................................49
- Stage 2: Balance ..................................................................................................55
    - Factors affecting the fertile state ..................................................................56
    - Beliefs, emotions and the body .....................................................................59
    - Approaches to create balance .......................................................................62
- Stage 3: Resolve ..................................................................................................89
    - The importance of resolution for fertility ....................................................91
    - Who is to blame? ...........................................................................................94
    - How to identify issues that may need to be resolved ..................................95
    - Some possible approaches for resolution ....................................................96
    - Some possible issues to resolve ....................................................................98
    - Some possible areas of inner conflict ..........................................................98
    - Unconscious blocks .......................................................................................99
    - Age .................................................................................................................103
    - Previous termination ...................................................................................105
    - Miscarriage ...................................................................................................108
    - Stillbirth and neonatal death ......................................................................114
    - Menstrual health ..........................................................................................115
    - Parenthood ...................................................................................................123
- Stage 4: Enhance ................................................................................................125
    - Visualisation approaches to enhance fertility ............................................126
    - Considerations when working with visualisation approaches .................127
    - The applications of visualisation approaches for fertility .........................129
    - Visualisation scripts to enhance fertility ....................................................132
    - Working with physical problems to enhance fertility ...............................133
- Stage 5: Prepare .................................................................................................137
    - Preparation for pregnancy ..........................................................................138
    - Preparation for birth ...................................................................................143

  Preparation for parenthood .................................................. 149
  Preparation for medical treatments .................................... 154
Stage 6: Support ..................................................................................... 157
  Support to maintain change .................................................. 158
  How to maintain change ........................................................ 159
  The importance of emotional support ................................. 162
  Support during pregnancy .................................................... 163
  Support after miscarriage and stillbirth ............................. 164
  IVF and other medical treatment failure ........................... 165
  Choosing not to become parents .......................................... 167
  Looking at the options for parenthood .............................. 171
  Moving on ................................................................................. 173
Working with men ................................................................................ 177

## Stage 1: Outcome

The first stage of the *Fertile Body Method* is to determine what outcome the client wants from therapy. *Stage 1: Outcome* is possibly the most important part of the *Fertile Body Method* during which we identify the client's goal for therapy, gather information, build rapport, and create a treatment plan.

For those who are unfamiliar with effective goal-setting approaches, the following section contains detailed information about how to create good therapeutic goals using solution focused questions and techniques.

In this section I have also given a few examples of some of the basic educative information that you may need to share with your client to ensure that they understand hypnosis and the relationship between the mind and the body. A case study at the end of this section illustrates how the goal can be used, alongside the *Fertile Body Method* framework, to create a therapeutic treatment plan.

**This section contains:**
Set the goal:

- Goal setting
- Goal setting for fertility
- Managing expectations
- Essential steps to creating a goal
- Using the goal to create a therapeutic strategy
- A solution focused approach
- What is solution focused therapy?
- Questions for creating the goal
- Prioritising goals
- Working with scales
- Reviewing the changes between sessions.

Assess the information:

- Questionnaire
- GP diagnosis
- Taking a case history
- Assessing the information
- Selecting techniques
- Choosing appropriate homework
- Creating a therapeutic treatment plan.

Inform the client:

- About hypnotherapy
- The mind-body connection
- Fertility Awareness Education.

Case study:

- Assessing and creating a therapeutic treatment plan.

## Set the goal

*The law of floatation was not discovered by the contemplation of the sinking of things.*
                              Thomas Troward (1847–1916)

To work effectively with fertility problems we need to understand more about what it is we are working towards. An obvious starting point is to consider what fertility is and what it means to the client. Fertility is defined as: "Capable of initiating, sustaining, or supporting reproduction." (American Psychological Association, 2000)

I believe that when the mind and body are in a state of wellbeing, the body will naturally produce the conditions needed for reproduction. It seems that equilibrium and wellbeing are an important aspect of fertility and reproduction. We know however, that millions of people get pregnant and have babies when they are mentally, emotionally and physically unwell. So while overall wellbeing may not be necessary for fertility, it certainly seems that where there are problems, improving wellbeing and restoring balance can enhance fertility and increase the chances of having a baby. Although it is possible to work directly with the known causes of fertility problems, there is still so much that is unknown about fertility and so working towards improving psychological and physical health is more likely to address the 'unknown' causes.

In general terms, a fertile state is a state of mental, spiritual and physical balance which is experienced as a state of wellbeing. What this actually means to each individual will be an entirely unique thing. In order to understand what this means for a particular person we can ask them a series of questions. These questions, given later in this section, are designed to get specific and detailed information about what it will be like for them to be in a fertile state. This information is an essential part of the goal for therapy and will contain all the information you need about how to approach the ongoing treatment.

## Goal setting for fertility

*Contemplate yourself surrounded by the conditions you wish to create.*
                                                                Dr Wayne Dyer

With the treatment of any condition, the goal is vitally important. The goal needs to be realistic and achievable to ensure that the person will be capable of succeeding. A well-formed goal for therapy needs to be *SMART* and *healthy*.

- A *SMART goal* is one that is Specific, Measurable, Achievable, Realistic and Timely.

- A *healthy goal* is rational, flexible and consistent with reality.

Typically when someone comes to see me with fertility concerns they come with the implicit goal of having a baby. Certainly this is true in the majority of cases but there are of course those who come to see me with other goals, such as 'to lose weight/stop smoking/stop drinking to improve fertility', 'to reduce stress/stop worrying', 'to deal with fear of hospitals/birth/parenthood', and so on.

When I first started working in the field of fertility and clients came to see me 'to have a baby' I found myself feeling unusually stressed and pressurised. Something didn't seem quite right to me, until one day I realised that we were working towards a goal that neither I nor they had any 'control' over.

'Having a baby' is neither a SMART nor healthy goal since it is not necessarily achievable. By achievable, I mean that the person is likely to reach the outcome if they fulfil certain criteria, follow certain steps and take certain actions. Part of the challenge of fertility problems is that having a baby can never be guaranteed, and may not necessarily result, even if all the 'correct' and appropriate steps are taken.

## Managing expectations

If 'having a baby' is not a suitable goal for therapy, what is? How can we manage the client's expectation that by seeing you, they will conceive and have a baby?

Although often the person has come to you with the sole motivation of having a baby, an important part of the therapeutic process involves creating this goal in a SMART healthy way, helping them recognise that the goal of having a baby might be counterproductive. To aim to achieve something that ultimately may not happen will lead to stress, anxiety, hopelessness and potential failure.

It is important, therefore, to separate the intention from the goal. Intention is a hope and a desired outcome whereas the goal must be something that can be worked towards and achieved; it should help to make the couple's intention to have a baby far more likely.

Making the distinction between intention and goal not only ensures that both you and the client are working towards something that is obtainable but minimises the likelihood of false expectations, disappointment and further feelings of hopelessness.

## The essential steps to creating a SMART healthy goal

1. First explain to the client that a SMART and healthy goal will have all the following qualities:
    - A SMART goal will be: Specific, Measurable, Achievable, Realistic and Timely.
    - A healthy goal will be: rational, flexible and consistent with reality.

2. Explain how 'getting pregnant or having a baby' is neither SMART nor healthy since it is not achievable (in the sense that they can't control it or make it happen) and nor is it flexible. Having a goal that doesn't have specific steps towards attaining it will create unnecessary stress and set them up for potential failure.

3. Reassure them that they can, of course, hold on to their intention to have children, and in fact the best way of increasing the likelihood of that intention being achieved is by creating a goal that will support it. Their current goal of having children is in some ways counterproductive and only adds to feelings of stress and feeling 'out of control'.

   *For example: I understand that what you really want is to conceive and give birth to a healthy, beautiful baby. It's important that you hold that intention as your ultimate outcome, however, in order for us to work together effectively we need to create a goal that is SMART. A SMART goal is a goal that is Specific, Measurable, Achievable (there are steps that you can take that will allow you to achieve it), Realistic and Timely. As you know, the goal of having a baby is not something that can be guaranteed, even if you take specific steps towards it. But we also know that there are all kinds of things that will certainly help you move towards that, but unfortunately having a baby is one of those things that really isn't up to us. It's part of the great mystery of life, as to when and how and who will get pregnant. So I guess it's fair to say that having a baby in some ways is not a 'realistic' goal. In fact the best way to support your intention to have a baby is to create a goal that is SMART and will help you create the best possible conditions for pregnancy and birth. So I'd like to recommend that we look at creating a goal that will help you and your partner to be in an optimum fertile state. Would that be useful for you?*

4. Educate them about the effects of stress on the hormonal system (please refer to *Stage 2: Balance* for this explanation, Page 66). Explain how having a SMART and healthy goal can help reduce stress.

5. Ask questions that will help them consider what goal is most likely to enhance their chances of conceiving. For example:
   - To give yourself the best possible chance of conceiving, what changes do you need to make?
   - In order to conceive, you need to be in a fertile state. What would being in a fertile state mean for you?

These questions will direct their focus towards promoting the best possible circumstances which themselves will support fertility. In order to create a clear and well-defined goal, we would need to continue this line of questioning in a solution focused way. Please refer to the *Solution Focused Therapy* (Page 31) and *Questions for creating the goal* (Page 31) sections for a full description.

Many people know what a healthy fertile state is, and are able to identify what needs to change in order for them to move into this state. There are, however, many other people who haven't any prior knowledge of what this mental, emotional and physical health is like. In these cases it is useful to use analogies and metaphors to help them recognise what a harmonious and balanced state of health and fertility would be like.

## Take a solution focused approach

We know that the unconscious mind needs a clear message about what we want. The more detailed and specific this message is, the more easily the change can happen.

A solution focused approach is an effective way to convert abstract goals such as 'I want to be happy' into measurable and concrete goals: 'When I am happy, I will be smiling or laughing when I talk to my husband. When I walk to work I'll catch myself whistling and I'll also get back into my painting and drawing.'

Identifying these changes allows the client to know when things are happening that tell them they are making progress and when they have reached their goal. Solution focused questioning is an extremely effective means of creating a goal, ascertaining the steps you need to take to reach it, measuring progress and recognising when the goal has been achieved.

## Solution Focused Therapy (SFT)

The specific steps involved in its practice come from husband and wife Steve de Shazer and Insoo Kim Berg and their team at the Brief Family Therapy Family Center in Milwaukee, USA.

- Solution focused therapy (SFT) is a talking therapy that *focuses on what clients want to achieve through therapy* rather than on the problem that made them seek help.

- It is an approach to psychotherapy based on *solution-building* rather than problem-solving.

- It explores *current resources and future hopes* rather than present problems and past causes.

- Solution focused therapy helps people *identify the things that they wish to change in their life* and also *to attend to those things that are currently happening that they wish to continue happening*.

- It helps people construct a *concrete vision of a preferred future* for themselves. It then identifies times in their current life that are closer to this future, and examines what is different on these occasions.

- By bringing these *small successes to their awareness*, and helping them repeat the successful things they do when the problem is not there or less severe, the therapist helps the client move towards the preferred future they have identified.

## Questions for creating the goal

The following solution focused questions can help create a clear, concrete and observable goal that can be measured and, when it is achieved, will be obvious to both the therapist and the client.

*Before the session, on the telephone*

Asking the client to give some thought to their goals for therapy before they come to see you is a very good way of setting the change in motion. It also gives the client time to think it through and clarify their intention. Sometimes this pre-appointment process alone can make a big difference to how the client feels by the time they come to see you.

> *Before you come and see me it would be useful if you could spend some time clarifying what you want to get out of this treatment. Ask yourself what changes you want to make. How will you be thinking, feeling and behaving as a result of these changes? Try to be as specific as possible. Say what you want rather than what you don't want. I would recommend you write it all down and bring it with you when you come for your appointment.*

### Questions to create a preferred future

The following are examples of questions that will help the client identify what changes they want to make in their life. These questions are not necessarily specific to fertility but will help clarify the changes the client needs to make if they are to improve their general health and wellbeing.

- What changes would you like to see as a result of our time together?
- If coming to see me was useful to you, how would you know?
- If you weren't going through any of the problems that you are going through now, how would your life be different?
- What are your best hopes for coming to see me?
- And how will things be different for you when all of that (best hopes) is happening?
- How will those changes show themselves to the people around you?
- How will those changes be good for you?
- How will you know that?
- What else will tell you?

### Questions to create a fertile state

The following are examples of solution focused questions that can help the client determine what a fertile state would be like for them.

- How would you describe a state of fertility and health?

- What do you think will help you to have a baby?

- What else? (repeat x 10)

- What things are already in place?

- When you are in a state of mental, emotional and physical balance, how will you know?

- How else? (repeat x 20)

- What changes will you notice in the way you think?

- What changes will you notice in the way you feel?

- What changes will you notice in the way you behave?

- Who would be the first to notice these changes?

- How will these changes affect those around you? Friends, family, colleagues and partner?

- How will these changes affect your work? Your social life? Your home?

- When you are in a fertile state, how will you know?

- What will you be doing differently?

- How will you be thinking?

- How will you be feeling?

- How will your body be responding?

- And how will things be different for you when all of that is happening?

- How will those changes show themselves to the people around you?

- How will those changes be good for you?

- How will you know that?

- What differences will that make?

Repeating the questions 'how else' and 'what else', as indicated above, will help the client widen their answers with further examples and ways in which the change may happen.

*Techniques for describing the goal state*

When asking questions to determine the goal state, the following techniques can be useful:

- To get a positive statement, ask instead?
  *When you are not feeling so anxious, how will you be feeling instead?*

- Ask questions that elicit concrete and observable information
  *How will that show?*
  *How will you know?*

- Get answers that are detailed
  *What specifically will change when you have more perspective on this situation?*

- Get multiple perspectives
  *What will your best friend notice about you when you are feeling more relaxed?*

- Consider the changes in relationships
  *How will that change positively affect your relationship with your husband/wife?*

- Ask about interactions
  *How will s/he respond differently to you?*

- Enquire about change in different contexts: work, home, friends, social events
  *When you are feeling more confident, how will that show at work?*

- Find out more about it
  *So when you feel more relaxed you say you will notice it most by the way you talk to your husband more calmly. What else will you notice when you feel more relaxed? What else? What else?*

- Look for the first tiny signs
  *What will be the first tiny signs that will indicate that you are moving towards this healthy fertile state?*

## Prioritising goals

Through solution focused questions you can establish the overall goal state for therapy. The goal may consist of different aspects or it is possible that the client may have a few very different goals for therapy. It is important to prioritise the goals so that it is clear which needs to be addressed first. The simplest way to do this is to ask the client, 'Looking at these changes you want to make, which of them is the most important to you?'

The priority of goals may also indicate the therapeutic priorities. In some cases though, the goal priorities may be different to the therapeutic priorities and it may be necessary to make one particular change before tackling another issue. A good example of this may be where the client has experienced a birth trauma.

The client's priorities may be to first resolve the trauma then develop enough strength to cope and finally to be ready to try for another baby. In this case the therapist needs to consider that safe and effective practice means that emotional stability should be achieved before any trauma work can be done. It follows that once the client has access to their inner resources and has cleared the effect that the trauma is still having on their life now, they will indeed be more ready to try for another baby.

In the above example, the *Fertile Body Method* offers a guide for prioritising and creating a safe and effective therapeutic strategy. Once the outcome (Stage 1) has been determined, balance and emotional stability (Stage 2) need to be established before moving on to resolving (Stage 3) the traumatic birth.

Another way to assess the priority of different goals is by using scaling. The section below titled *Working with scales* gives some further examples of this.

## Working with scales

Scaling questions can be used to identify useful differences for the client and practitioner and may help them establish goals and to gauge change and progress in the follow-up sessions.

One of the most useful frameworks for a solution focused interview is the 0 to 10 scale, where 10 equals the achievement of all goals and 0 is the worst possible scenario.

Scales can also be used to differentiate between different aspects of the problem and its solution. For example, a person with depression might feel anxious and demotivated. Both of these aspects might be explored through separate scales. Similarly, when the client is experiencing multiple problems, each problem can be assessed with its own scale.

The goals and solutions that the client is moving towards can be set on a scale from 0 to 10, while disturbance and difficulty can be scaled from -10 to 0. This creates a continuum scale that is always directed upwards.

The disturbance and difficulty scale is useful for:

- how much a particular past event is disturbing them now
- gauging how much they believe an unhealthy belief
- rating negative unhealthy emotions
- determining the priority of a particular issue.

Priority can be given to the problems that are scaled the highest when asked 'On a scale of -10 to 0 where -10 represents the greatest disturbance and 0 represents no disturbance at all, how much does that bother you now?'

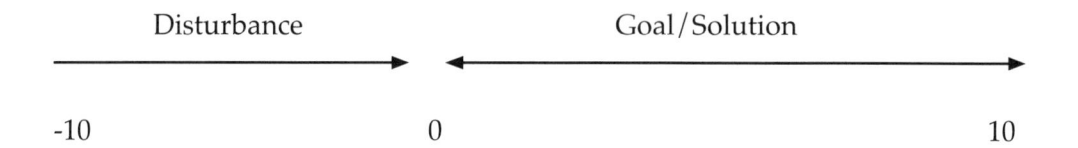

```
        Disturbance              Goal/Solution
   ─────────────────────▶   ◀─────────────────────▶

  -10                       0                       10
```

## Scaling technique and questions

- Set up the scale and assign 10 to the goal and 0 to the worst it has ever been.
  *10 stands for everything that you hope for from our talking together is happening, and 0 stands for none of it, not even the tiniest little bit of it is happening at present.*

- Ask the client to rate their current position on the scale.
  *Where now?*
  *What tells you that you are there and not at 0?*
  *What else tells you? (Repeat x 10)*

- Use questions to help the client identify resources.
  *What's stopping you from slipping one point lower down the scale?*
  *How have you managed to be at this level with everything that's been going on?*

- Use questions to help the client identify exceptions.
  *On a day when you are one point higher on the scale, what would tell you that it was a 'one point higher' day?*
  *How will you know that you have moved one point up?*
  *How else? (Repeat x 10)*

- Use questions to help the client describe a preferred future.
  *Where on the scale would be good enough? What would a day at that point on the scale look like?*

## *Using scales to review the changes between sessions*

Scales can be used as a way to review the changes between sessions and ask questions that will encourage the client to recognise what is different since the last session. Scaling provides a concrete and specific way of identifying change and being able to recognise when a goal has been achieved.

- Remind the client of the scale which was created.
  *I want you to recall that scale we created at the last session where 10 stands for \_\_\_\_\_ (insert the client's goal) and 0 stands for none of it, not even the tiniest little bit of it is happening at present.*

- Ask the client to rate their current position on the scale.
  *Where are you on that scale now?*
  *What tells you that you are there and not at 0?*
  *What else tells you? (Repeat x 10)*

- If they have gone down on the scale since the last session.
  *How have you managed to keep yourself from slipping down any lower on that scale?*
  *What did that take?*

- Use questions to help the client describe the next step.
  *If you were to move another point up that scale, how would you know?*
  *When you have moved one more point up that scale, what will your husband notice has changed?*

## Assess the information

### Questionnaire

The questionnaire is a document containing all the relevant questions regarding the couple's lifestyle, fertility and medical history. The questionnaire (a copy can be downloaded from the CD) can be sent out to the client before their appointment which will give them enough time to find any information regarding their medical history which they don't have available at their fingertips. Receiving a completed questionnaire before the start of the session can also save time during the initial consultation.

| **QUESTIONNAIRE FOR WOMEN** |
|---|
| **Personal Details** |
| Name |
| Address |
|  |
| Telephone |
| Email |
| Date of birth |
| Age |
| Occupation |
| Partner's name |
| Marital status |
| How long have you been together? |
|  |
|  |
| **Medical Practitioners** |
| Doctor (GP) |
|     Name |
|     Address |
|  |
|     Telephone |
| Fertility Clinic |

## QUESTIONNAIRE FOR WOMEN *(contd)*

| | |
|---|---|
| Clinic name | |
| Consultant's name | |

**Fertility History**

Have you seen your GP about your fertility?

What diagnosis did you receive?

How long have you been trying for a baby?

Have you ever been pregnant?

Have you ever experienced a miscarriage?

If yes, please provide details of when and at what stage of pregnancy.

Do you or your partner have any children?

Please give details such as name and age.

Have you ever terminated a pregnancy?

Is this termination confidential?

What tests and investigations have you had? e.g. FSH, progesterone, scans

What medical treatments have you had for fertility? e.g. IUI, Comid, IVF

| Date | Treatment | Clinic | Outcome |
|---|---|---|---|
| | | | |
| | | | |
| | | | |
| | | | |
| | | | |
| | | | |
| | | | |

## QUESTIONNAIRE FOR WOMEN (contd)

*What complementary treatments have you had for fertility? e.g. acupuncture*

### Menstrual Health

*Have you ever used any form of contraception?*
*What, and for how long?*

*At what age did you start your periods?*
*What was this experience like for you?*

*Have you ever experienced irregular cycles?*
*Currently, how long is each cycle?*
*How many days is your period?*
*Are they light, average or heavy?*
*Are your periods ever painful?*
*Do you experience any premenstrual symptoms?*
*Details*

*Do you use tampons, sanitary pads, moon cup or other?*
*Do you ovulate every month?*
*How do you know that you are ovulating?*
*Are you aware of your fertile time?*
*Do you monitor your cervical mucus secretions?*

### General Health

*Weight*
*Height*

| **QUESTIONNAIRE FOR WOMEN** | *(contd)* |
|---|---|
| Do you / have you been diagnosed with: | |
|     PCOS ☐ | |
|     Endometriosis ☐ | |
|     Fibroids ☐ | |
|     Gynaecological problems ☐ | |
| What health problems have you had in the past? | |
| What health problems are you still experiencing? | |
| Are you taking any medication? | |
| Are you taking any other supplements, remedies or herbs? | |
| ***Sexual Relationship*** | |
| Do you experience any difficulties in your sexual relationship? | |
| Has trying for a baby affected your sex life? | |
| How frequently do you have sex? | |
| ***Family History*** | |
| Is there any history of fertility problems in your family? | |
| Is there any history of miscarriage? | |
| Is there any history of birth trauma? | |
| Are your parents still alive? | |
| Are your parents still married? | |
| How many brothers and sisters do you have? | |
| What is your position in the family? (e.g. oldest, middle, 4th) | |
| Do any of your siblings have children? | |

## QUESTIONNAIRE FOR WOMEN (contd)

### Mental Health

| |
|---|
| Have you ever suffered from depression? |
| Have you ever suffered from any psychiatric condition? |
| Have you ever struggled with addiction? |
| |
| |

### Lifestyle

| |
|---|
| How many hours do you sleep on average per night? |
| Do you exercise? |
| Details |
| |
| What is your diet like? |
| Have you seen a nutritionist? |
| Do you smoke? |
| Do you take any recreational drugs? |
| How many hours a week do you work? |
| How much time do you spend commuting every day? |
| What are your interests and hobbies? |
| |
| |
| What else do you do to relax? |
| |
| |

## QUESTIONNAIRE FOR MEN

### Personal Details

| |
|---|
| Name |
| Address |
| |
| Telephone |
| Email |

# The Stages of Treatment

| **QUESTIONNAIRE FOR MEN** |
|---|
| Date of birth |
| Age |
| Occupation |
| Partner's name |
| Marital status |
| How long have you been together? |
| |
| **Medical Practitioners** |
| Doctor (GP) |
|     Name |
|     Address |
| |
|     Telephone |
| |
| Fertility Clinic |
|     Clinic name |
|     Consultant's name |
| |
| **Fertility History** |
| How long have you been trying for a baby? |
| Have you ever conceived with another partner? |
| Do you or your partner have any children? |
| Please give details such as name and age. |
| |
| What tests and investigations have you had? e.g. sperm test, male hormone |
| |
| |
| |
| |
| Have you ever had a vasectomy? |
| |

| **QUESTIONNAIRE FOR MEN** | *(contd)* |
|---|---|
| *What fertility treatments have you had?* | |
| | |
| *What complementary treatments have you had for fertility?* | |
| | |
| **General Health** | |
| Weight | |
| Height | |
| What health problems have you had in the past? | |
| | |
| What health problems are you still experiencing? | |
| | |
| Are you taking any medication? | |
| | |
| Are you taking any other supplements, remedies or herbs? | |
| | |
| **Sexual Relationship** | |
| Do you experience any difficulties in your sexual relationship? | |
| | |
| Has trying for a baby affected your sex life? | |
| | |
| Do you have any difficulties getting or maintaining an erection? | |
| | |
| Do you have a low sex drive? | |
| How frequently do you have sex? | |
| | |
| **Family History** | |
| Is there any history of fertility problems in your family? | |
| Is there any history of miscarriage? | |
| Is there any history of birth trauma? | |
| Are your parents still alive? | |
| Are your parents still married? | |
| How many brothers and sisters do you have? | |

| **QUESTIONNAIRE FOR MEN** | *(contd)* |
|---|---|
| *What is your position in the family? (e.g. oldest, middle, 4th)* | |
| *Do any of your siblings have children?* | |
| | |
| **Mental Health** | |
| *Have you ever suffered from depression?* | |
| *Have you ever suffered from any psychiatric condition?* | |
| *Have you ever struggled with addiction?* | |
| | |
| **Lifestyle** | |
| *How many hours do you sleep on average per night?* | |
| *Do you exercise?* | |
| *Details* | |
| *What is your diet like?* | |
| *Have you seen a nutritionist?* | |
| *Do you smoke?* | |
| *Do you take hot baths or saunas?* | |
| *Do you wear tight fitting clothing?* | |
| *Do you take any recreational drugs?* | |
| *How many hours a week do you work?* | |
| *How much time do you spend commuting every day?* | |
| *What are your interests and hobbies?* | |
| | |
| *What else do you do to relax?* | |
| | |
| | |
| | |

## GP diagnosis

If someone has come to see you with concerns about their fertility or related issues, you would need to ask them if they have been to see their doctor and/or specialist. It is generally recommended that couples trying for a baby should visit their GP if they aren't pregnant after one year of regular unprotected sex (if they are under the age of 35) or after six months if they are over 35.

In some cases it is best not to wait for this period of time. People should consider seeing their doctor earlier if:

- They are over 38
- They have had a previous ectopic pregnancy or more than one miscarriage
- Have had any sexually transmitted disease
- Experience pain during intercourse
- The woman's periods are painful, have stopped or are irregular
- The man has had any previous trauma to the testicles or had undescended testicles as a small boy
- The man suffers from premature ejaculation.

## Taking a case history

The goal setting process using solution focused questions will provide you with a clear idea of the goal for therapy while the questionnaire will give you all the necessary medical information as well as specific background information that is relevant to the couple's fertility.

The case history should be aimed at gathering information about the client's background and the events that have led to their current situation. The following question will encourage the client to consider what issues throughout their life could be relevant to their current situation.

*Case history question:*

> *Please tell me about your life, from birth to now. Please give me an overview, highlighting anything that you think is relevant to your current situation.*

I would then recommend spending some time going through the questionnaire, making further enquiries about anything that raises any questions.

The case history is an opportunity to get a fuller picture of the client's current situation. As they are answering questions, it is helpful to take note of their body language and other non-verbal cues, as this can provide information about what impact their past experiences are having on them now.

Throughout the case history scales can be used to check how much past experiences are disturbing them now and to determine the key issues and priorities for treatment.

*Scaling question*

> *On a scale from -10 to 0, where -10 represents the greatest disturbance and 0 represents no disturbance at all, how much are you affected by your mother's death now?*

## Assessing the information to determine the therapeutic strategy

A well-formed goal will inform your therapeutic strategy. The goal provides a picture of the outcome or destination that the client is moving towards and the specific information about how they will know when they get there will provide a direction and a map to the destination.

In addition to the agreed goal, the therapeutic strategy is determined by taking into account information from the:

- Questionnaire
- Case History
- Scales and priorities

# The Fertile Body Method

- Observed non-verbal information: body language, voice, facial expressions

- Client's predominant modality: are they visual, auditory or kinaesthetic

- Your own therapeutic intuition: the information that you unconsciously receive about your client combined with your own experience and inner wisdom.

During the initial consultation and throughout therapy it is useful to make notes of certain information about the client. These observations will help to highlight things that can be used to tailor the treatment and make use of the client's resources in the best possible way. The following information about the client may be useful to note:

- Strengths and interests

- Internal and external resources needed

- Previous experience with fertility and/or birth

- Expectations of therapy and expectations for change

- Belief system

- Current condition

- Time scales and financial resources

- Contraindications.

Once the goal, questionnaire and additional information have been noted and assessed, you can then use the six stages of the *Fertile Body Method* to help you create an effective treatment plan. Having completed *Stage 1: Outcome* of this approach, you can then consider which will be the most relevant stages of treatment to include in the treatment plan. You will find more information about each stage in the following chapters.

A treatment plan serves as a guide for therapy and will provide focus and direction to the treatment. It is important however to be flexible with the treatment plan so that it can change from session to session depending on the client's feedback and progress.

## The Stages of Treatment

*Using the goal to create a therapeutic strategy*

Essentially, a SMART and healthy goal will emphasise the positive changes that being in a healthy, fertile state will bring and will also include specific information about what that will mean for the client. The specific details about the fertile state as given by the client will hold the key to your therapeutic approach. The information will indicate what steps need to be taken as well as the thoughts, feelings and behaviours that would need to change in order to be in this state. In other words, a well-formed, detailed goal state will not only provide information about the destination, it will also give you the map and the directions needed to get there. This is illustrated in the case study at the end of this chapter (Page 52).

## Inform the client

The following is an example of an explanation that can be given to the client about hypnotherapy, the mind-body connection and the effect of unhealthy negative emotions on fertility. This is an important part of therapy since it empowers the client with knowledge and understanding and builds trust and rapport. I have also included some information here about Fertility Awareness Education, as it may be necessary to ensure that the couple are having intercourse at the right time. An overwhelming number of people are uninformed or have inaccurate information about when they are fertile and able to conceive.

### About Hypnotherapy

*Hypnosis is a natural state that you go in and out of every day. Each night, as you are falling asleep, when your body starts to feel relaxed and your mind begins to drift deeper into your own inner world, you are entering the hypnogogic state. You are not fully awake nor are you asleep since you are aware of things around you and yet you are giving all of your attention to your own inner thoughts and feelings.*

*This natural trance state, which you also experience when you become absorbed in any activity, is a very good state for absorbing new learning. When you enter this trance state for therapeutic benefit, your heartrate and breathing slow down as you access what is known as the relaxation response. The relaxation response produces a state that helps counteract the negative effects of stress on the body. So simply being in this state of deep relaxation is highly beneficial.*

*In this hypnotic state your conscious mind is less 'active' allowing you to have greater access to your own unconscious resources and innate wisdom.*

*The unconscious mind is pre-verbal. While language is a tool for the conscious mind, the unconscious mind stores information in symbols, patterns and images. In a state of hypnosis we often use visualisation, symbols, patterns and metaphor to help create change on an unconscious level.*

## The mind-body connection

*Your mind and body are in constant communication with each other. Every thought you have produces a chemical change in your body. Some experiential examples of this occur when you think about something that terrifies you and you experience physical sensations such as 'butterflies' in your stomach. If you imagine someone whom you find very attractive caressing and kissing you, you might notice a warmth or tingling sensation in your body.*

*It is especially important to be aware of how negative unhealthy thoughts and emotions affect your body and your health. If you have ever been through a period of intense worry and stress you will have noticed how you lacked energy and vitality and your physical health deteriorated. When we experience emotions, hormones (chemical messengers) are released into our body. After prolonged periods of experiencing unhealthy emotions such as anxiety, the body's natural hormonal balance becomes disturbed. For example, excessive stress may lead to complete suppression of the menstrual cycle, and in less severe cases will lead to anovulation or irregular menstrual cycles. In order to create change to your health and fertility, your thoughts and emotional responses need to be healthy, too.*

## Fertility Awareness Education

Fertility Awareness Education teaches women a natural method that involves charting three primary fertility signs on a daily basis so their fertility can be accurately determined. Fertility awareness can help couples maximise their chances of conception by recognising signs of fertility and optimising the timing of intercourse.

*What is fertility awareness?*

- Understanding basic information about fertility and reproduction
- Identifying the signs and symptoms of fertility during the woman's fertility cycle
- Recognising the changes in a woman's fertility cycle
- Understanding ovulation and the viability of the egg
- Understanding that sperm are viable for a number of days in optimum conditions
- Using this knowledge to plan or avoid pregnancy and control fertility.

The questionnaire may indicate that the client is unaware of her fertile times, and possibly isn't too aware of her menstrual cycle. Generally this is not the case with people who have been having problems conceiving for a long time, and more often than not they know everything that there is to know about fertility. Some women use ovulation kits and thermometers to track their ovulation. While this can be useful in some cases, it can also add to stress. If a woman is using a kit or taking her temperature every day it may distract her from paying attention to the natural physical and emotional signs of fertility and can make trying for a baby very mechanical.

It may be healthier to encourage the client to become more sensitive to her cycle so that she can notice the natural rise in libido during her fertile time. This may lead to sexual intercourse being the result of increased desire rather than a change in basal body temperature.

For those who are not aware of their fertile time, it is necessary to inform them about the changes that happen in their body during the different phases of their cycle and that intercourse needs to happen roughly between day seven and day fourteen (when day one is the first day of their period) of their cycle, depending on the length of their cycle. More specific information about Fertility Awareness Education and the menstrual cycle can be found in *How to determine the fertile time*, Section D of this book (Page 304), and a Fertile Awareness Education programme handout, can be downloaded from the CD to give to your clients.

> ### Case study: assessing and creating a treatment plan
>
> To illustrate an approach to creating a treatment plan I would like to highlight the goal from a client's case history. Samantha's goal for therapy is to prepare herself mentally, emotionally and physically so that she can conceive naturally. She has been trying to conceive for the past year, and has been diagnosed with unexplained infertility.
>
> Following a series of solution focused questions, she created a clear picture of what this goal meant to her, and how she would know when she had reached it:
>
>> *When I am mentally prepared to conceive I will be calmer and my mind will be a lot clearer. I will know this has happened because when I am at home in the evening I will be sitting quietly on the sofa, probably reading a good book. I will be able to concentrate and focus completely on the book that I am reading. Generally I'll just be able to focus more on whatever it is I am doing instead of being distracted by 'What if's' and 'Why me?' and 'It's never going to happen'. When I am calmer, I will know because I will be talking more slowly. My husband is likely to notice this because he always says I talk at 100 miles an hour and wonders how I manage to breathe. So I guess I will be breathing more deeply too. I will also be thinking that it is possible for me to get pregnant and that my body is capable of conceiving. When I really believe this I'll know because I won't be so affected when I see other pregnant women. Instead when I see them I will think, 'Yeah, that's probably what I'll look like sooner or later'. So I'll just generally be a bit more positive in my attitude.*
>>
>> *When I am ready and prepared emotionally I'll be more confident in myself. I'll be more confident in myself as a woman. I'll probably be more confident in my ability to cope as a mother. So I'll believe that I can be a good mother. I'll know that I have this confidence because when I picture myself with a baby I will see myself at ease and relaxed. But probably the most important way I will know that I am prepared is because I will be feeling relaxed. I'll notice this relaxation most in my body, because my shoulders will be loose and comfortable instead of being tensed up next to my ears. All of this will make such a difference to my life because I will be able to enjoy things more. When I feel more relaxed I'm probably going to have more fun and laughter, like I used to when I met up with my friends. So my friends will notice this relaxation because I'll be joking around again and laughing.*

## The Stages of Treatment

> *When my body is prepared I'll be about several pounds lighter. I'll be stronger too. I'll be doing yoga three times a week. This will make me feel really good about myself because I'll feel much lighter and more flexible too. I'll know that I'm at this point because when I walk into my kitchen I will see the fruit and vegetable rack overflowing with brightly coloured foods.*

The details of this goal indicate what the main emphasis of change needs to be.

- Calmness and concentration – reduce worry, 'What if's' and 'Why me?' etc.

- Relaxation – 'more fun and laughter' and 'shoulders will be loose' and 'breathing more deeply'

- Confidence – 'It is possible for me to get pregnant' and 'I'll believe that I can be a good mother'

- Exercise and diet – 'doing yoga' and 'fruit and vegetable rack overflowing'.

This information should be considered in relation to the stages of treatment – Balance, Resolve, Enhance, Prepare, Support.

In this particular case study, the next step of the treatment should be focused on creating relaxation by reducing stress and worry/unhealthy beliefs and making healthy changes to Samantha's diet and increasing her exercise. Once Samantha is feeling more relaxed it may be necessary to resolve some issues which could be contributing to the lack of confidence in her ability to be a mother. Her natural fertility can be enhanced through visualisation focused on seeing herself as a mother coping calmly and easily. Homework can be given to help her feel more prepared for parenthood. And finally to support her to maintain this healthy attitude and the lifestyle changes in the months ahead.

## *Based on the goal, the treatment plan for Samantha could be:*

Stage 2: Balance

- Reduce stress and worry
- Address unhealthy beliefs
- Changes to diet.

- Increase exercise

Stage 3: Resolve

- Identify issues affecting confidence about being a mother
- Resolve past events to increase confidence in self as a mother

Stage 5: Prepare

- Prepare for parenthood

Stage 6: Support

- Support to maintain lifestyle changes
- Support to maintain levels of relaxation
- Support to maintain a healthy attitude.

## *Stage 2: Balance*

The second stage of the *Fertile Body Method* is designed to create emotional stability, balance and to build inner resources. This section describes the factors that affect fertility and how beliefs and emotions affect the body. Discussions and approaches for creating mental, emotional and physical balance are included, as well as suggestions about how to increase the client's access to the inner resources that may be needed to achieve the therapeutic goal.

Along with *Stage 1: Outcome*, this stage provides some of the vital and necessary ingredients for change. I consider this stage to be essential for safely and effectively resolving any issues that may need to be addressed in *Stage 3: Resolve*, since it ensures that the client is in a receptive and resourceful state to be able to deal with any potentially disturbing issues that may arise.

**This section contains:**
**Factors affecting the fertile state:**

- Internal factors
- External factors
- The importance of having our physical and emotional needs met.

**Beliefs, emotions and the body:**

- What are unhealthy beliefs?
- How unhealthy beliefs affect our emotions and body
- How unhealthy beliefs affect fertility.

**Approaches to create balance:**

- Create balance – overview
- General health
- Diet
- Lifestyle (work, smoking, alcohol, drugs, etc.)
- Emotional states (stress, depression, fear, anxiety)
- Beliefs (unhealthy beliefs and unconscious blocks)

- Physical symptoms (PCOS, endometriosis, low sperm count) and hormonal balance (high follicle stimulating hormone levels, etc.)

- Relationship issues

- Spiritual beliefs

- Inner resources.

## *Factors affecting the fertile state*

*It is invariably a combination of both external and internal causes that creates illness, rather than just one cause on its own. This is important to remember, as healing almost always comes through the combination of both physical and psycho/emotional therapeutic work.*

(Shapiro, 2008, p. 30)

In order to have a baby, each partners' body needs to be working effectively so that the necessary sperm and eggs can be produced, fertilised, implanted, developed and birthed. This complicated and miraculous process can be interrupted and affected by a wide variety of factors, only some of which we know how to consciously alter and control.

I have divided the factors that affect fertility into internal and external factors. Many people are well aware of how external factors such as diet and environment affect fertility but are less aware of the impact of the internal factors on fertility. Scientific research shows how the body and mind continuously influence and affect each other. This information, which is further explained later in this section (Page 57), can help us understand how fertility is more than just a physical state and can be affected and enhanced by changes in thinking and feeling.

Our body is a homeostatic system that aims to self-correct and rebalance unless it is prevented from doing so. Ongoing exposure to any of the negative external or internal factors can affect the natural balance in the body in such a way that fertility can be negatively impacted. Equally, if our basic emotional and physical needs are not being met, this too can lead to mental, emotional and physical disruptions. In this section we will further explore the ways in which the internal factors may affect fertility.

There are many different options to help restore mind-body balance. For this reason I suggest a few different ways to focus your approach. The method you choose to use will depend very much on the emphasis of the client's unique situation. For example, you may want to teach those clients who feel particularly disempowered, hopeless or out of control a selection of self-help tools they can use to support them through this experience. A person presenting with high levels of stress, anxiety and/or panic attacks would benefit most from treatment focused on promoting the relaxation response and rebalancing the autonomic nervous system.

However, other important therapeutic components should also be included. For example: treating high stress and anxiety by inducing the relaxation response and addressing the unhealthy beliefs that are responsible for maintaining that response. These different focuses of treatment are, therefore, really intended as a useful starting point but should then go on to include all the other necessary components for maintaining balance and helping to restore fertility.

## *The external and internal factors that affect fertility*

| External factors |
| --- |
| • Diet |
| • Environment |
| • Lifestyle |
| • Physical problems |
| • Age |

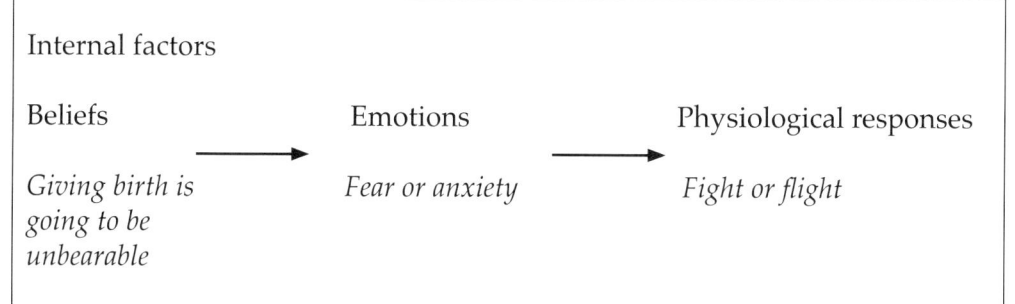

Internal factors

| Beliefs | Emotions | Physiological responses |
| --- | --- | --- |
| *Giving birth is going to be unbearable* | *Fear or anxiety* | *Fight or flight* |

Unhealthy beliefs that result in unhealthy negative emotions will, over time, disturb the natural balance in the body which can negatively affect fertility.

## The importance of having our needs met: a Human Givens Approach

The Human Givens framework offers a revolutionary new organising idea, which is derived from the latest scientific understanding from neurobiology, psychology, ancient wisdom and original new insights. The Human Givens Approach grew out of the work of a group of psychologists and psychotherapists whose aim was to discover why some psychotherapy approaches appeared to work and others didn't.

The result was a synthesis of everything that can reliably be said to help human beings function well and be happy. It soon became known as the Human Givens Approach, after the scientifically well-established 'givens' of human nature.

### What are the Human Givens?

A human being is a sentient, living organism that depends upon nourishment from its environment in order to sustain life and grow. Without a direct connection to our environment we would die. To ensure that we have the capacity to receive what we need from our environment we have an innate guidance system or higher intelligence.

Imbalances in our system occur when our essential needs are not being met. These needs are both physical and emotional. Our physical needs demand that we are safe, nourished and protected from the harsh elements. Our emotional needs are for security, autonomy and control, emotional intimacy, to give and receive attention and to feel a part of a wider community. We have a basic need for self-esteem (earned by our competence and achievement) and an inherent need for meaning in our lives.

If these needs are not being met at any given time, we experience an imbalance which will ultimately lead to a state of mental, emotional and physical disease (Griffin and Tyrrell, 2004b). The Human Givens Approach as outlined above has had a strong influence on the *Fertile Body Method*. The importance of having our needs met is the cornerstone for enhancing fertility and coming to terms with infertility. Restoring balance in *Stage 2: Balance* includes ensuring that the client's physical and emotional needs are being met. Some approaches for doing this can be found in *Approaches to create balance* (Page 62).

## Beliefs, emotions and the body

*A basic emotion such as fear can be described as an abstract feeling or a tangible molecule of the hormone adrenaline. Without the feeling there is no hormone; without the hormone there is no feeling. The revolution we call mind-body medicine was based on this simple discovery; wherever thought goes, a chemical goes with it.*

(Chopra, 1994)

## What are unhealthy beliefs?

We acquire our beliefs from the experiences we have and from the people around us. While some of the beliefs we have learnt are healthy and beneficial, others may be unhealthy and affect us in a harmful way.

Unhealthy beliefs are ideas that we hold which are:

- Rigid or extreme
- Inconsistent with reality
- Illogical or nonsensical
- Likely to lead to dysfunctional consequences.

A common example of an unhealthy belief that a woman who has been having problems conceiving may hold is:

> *I absolutely have to have a baby, because if I don't my life will be pointless and not worth living.*

This belief is rigid and demands that she *must* have a baby. This is unrealistic and inconsistent with reality since we know that not every woman in the world *must* or will have a baby. She concludes that if she does not have a baby her life will be pointless and not worth living, which objectively is nonsensical since it is possible for her life to be worthwhile irrespective of whether she has children or not. The consequence of her holding this belief is likely to be anxiety and further behaviour that perpetuates this state.

Holding unhealthy beliefs about life's adversities has a number of effects. These beliefs can:

- Lead to unhealthy negative emotions
- Lead you to act in self-defeating ways
- Impair and impact on the way you subsequently think
- Negatively affect your physical health and fertility.

Information about how to work with unhealthy beliefs is available in the section *Approaches to create balance* (Page 62).

## How unhealthy beliefs affect our emotions

Emotions are a response to an internal or external event, and arise because of the section beliefs we hold.

If we hold an unhealthy belief about a situation we will experience the negative unhealthy emotions that arise as a result of these beliefs. In this way we are all responsible for the emotional responses that we experience. Knowing this gives us the capacity to change the way we feel by changing the beliefs we hold.

For example, if three people were gathered in a room, and they all had problems conceiving and didn't have any children, would they all be feeling the same way?

Person A may be relieved: 'At least I know we've tried. It probably wasn't meant to be. Now my husband and I are free to follow our passion for travelling.'
Person B may be angry: 'I should've insisted that we start trying years ago but my husband said it was too soon. If we'd started then I would definitely be pregnant!'
Person C may be depressed: 'It's never going to happen for us. Life seems pointless knowing that we are going to spend the rest of our lives alone.'

It is the belief that each person holds about their situation that gives rise to their emotional response and thinking.

Examples of unhealthy negative emotions:

- Anxiety
- Depression

- Unhealthy anger
- Unhealthy jealousy
- Unhealthy envy
- Shame
- Hurt
- Guilt.

To find out more about these emotions, further reading on Cognitive Behavioural Therapy is recommended; please refer to the recommended reading list in Section E (Page 351).

## *How unhealthy beliefs and emotions affect fertility*

In recent years, much research has been done on the relationship between the mind and the body. Candace Pert, scientist and author of *Molecules of Emotions*, has shown that thoughts and feelings create chemicals called neuropeptides which have receptor sites throughout the body.

> *Beliefs affect your biology. When we have a thought or a feeling or an emotion then, in our brains, we make a set of chemicals known as neuropeptides. There are receptors to these chemical messengers not only in brain cells but also in other parts of our body, for example, in the cells of the immune system which protect us from cancer and infectious disease and degenerative disorders.*
>
> (Pert, 1985)

A good example of how beliefs affect the body can be found by looking more closely at the stress response. The beliefs that a person holds will determine whether they perceive a situation to be stressful or not. 'Stress', or more accurately the fight-or-flight response, is the body's natural reaction to threat or danger. This response is part of our innate survival system that helps us fight or flee a situation that we perceive to be unsafe.

Any situation that we interpret as not being okay in some way will trigger this response to a greater or lesser degree. This can be taken one step further to saying that any situation or experience that we resist, fight or don't accept will trigger this response in some way.

In situations of ongoing stress, increased levels of stress hormones such as adrenaline and cortisol will affect the body's natural biochemical balance. Since the hypothalamus regulates both the stress response as well as the sex hormones, any imbalance in thinking (resulting from an unhealthy belief) and feeling (such as anxiety) can directly impact on the reproductive system. This is relevant in natural conception as well as assisted reproduction since both require a healthy response from the reproductive system.

Healthy beliefs, resulting in healthy thinking and healthy emotions can bring balance back to the body's hormonal system and enhance fertility.

## *Approaches to create balance*

In this section I will identify and suggest some of the ways in which we can help to create mental, emotional and physical balance. Each area contains an explanation, a step-by-step approach as well as a list of useful techniques and scripts. Descriptions and details of these techniques and scripts can be found in Section C (Page 181). The techniques listed are not a definitive list, but instead offer some ideas and suggestions that can be added to the tools you already use.

### *Create balance – overview*

It is essential that balance is re-established before moving on to other stages of treatment. Emotional balance needs to be established first because when we are in a state of high emotional arousal our capacity to reason and think clearly is diminished. If we decrease emotional arousal first the client will be able to think more clearly and use her capacity to reason more easily.

By establishing emotional balance and stability, the client is also more likely to be able to access their own inner resources and strengths. In an emotionally disturbed state access to one's resources becomes limited. Creating a stable resourceful state is vital especially if there are traumas and other difficult issues to be resolved at a later stage. Unless the client is stabilised it is potentially unsafe and not recommended to proceed with *Stage 3: Resolve*.

This stage of treatment creates the foundation for change, and in many cases will be all that is required. Once someone is in a relaxed and resourceful state they are more likely to go on and resolve the relevant issues themselves.

## General health

To restore general health the basics of diet, lifestyle, sleep and exercise need to be considered. If these important things are taken care of then a person's wellbeing is likely to improve and they will also be less vulnerable to stress and depression.

Since stress and depression are often associated with fertility problems, it is quite common to find that regular sleeping patterns are affected. Ongoing sleep disruption can affect mental, emotional and physical health.

In cases where the client is having difficulty falling asleep because of excessive stress and worry, the following techniques are recommended:

- *Self-Integration Dissociation*: to clear your inner world from any thoughts or feelings that may be preventing you from drifting into a deep and refreshing sleep.

- *Favourite Place*: to be practised as a *Self-Hypnosis* technique before going to sleep at night to induce relaxation.

- *Tune Into Your Body Clock*: to restore the natural rhythms of the body.

- Follow all other suggestions made for stress reduction.

In cases where the client is waking in the early hours of the morning, this may indicate possible depression. Since sleep disturbance is likely to be a symptom of the depression, the depression needs to be dealt with. Refer to the suggestions for working with depression. The following technique may also be useful:

- *Apposition Of Opposites*: to balance the natural rhythms of the body and induce a healthy night's sleep.

## Diet

A healthy balanced nutritious diet is necessary in order to establish balance in the body. It will help to ensure that the body is healthy enough to conceive and nourish a developing baby. A healthy diet can also maintain sperm production at optimum levels. Being under- or overweight can also affect fertility.

A good detoxification programme can be highly beneficial for increasing fertility whether trying naturally or with assistance. Couples who have already been through medical treatment and are considering pursuing further treatments might want to consider doing a thorough detoxification in order to cleanse their body from the toxins accumulated during medical interventions.

I recommend referring your client to a nutritionist who specialises in fertility problems and can help with creating a suitable diet or detox programme. For details of recommended nutritionists please see the Resources section on the Fertile Body website (www.thefertilebody.com).

## *Lifestyle*

Our lifestyle is characterised by the habits, behaviours, values and attitudes we adopt for living.

Creating balance in our lifestyle is about reducing the habits that cause harm to us and increasing the activities that increase wellbeing. This includes balancing the amount of time we spend working and resting.

Many women gain a lot of fulfilment from their work and find that working gives them a positive focus in their life. However, many others find their work can be demanding and stressful. Women who are working long hours in busy jobs will need to reduce their work in order to stabilise their nervous system.

The following lifestyle changes will have a positive effect on fertility:

- Stop smoking: smokers are 50% more likely to miscarry and men who smoke have a lower sperm count and a 20% decrease in sperm motility.

- Stop drinking alcohol: alcohol may affect fertility and sperm quality. Even moderate drinking (less than three units a day) will decrease the chances of conception.

- Eliminate drugs: cocaine constricts blood vessels and so can affect the placenta and cause menstrual irregularities. Marijuana lowers sperm count, decreases sperm motility and lowers testosterone in males.

- Reduce caffeine: caffeine increases the chances of miscarriage and may increase the risk of developing endometriosis.

- Avoid saunas: anything that raises the temperature of a man's testicles can decrease sperm production and motility.

- Exercise gently: some research has suggested that vigorous exercise (raising heart rate over 110 beats per minute) may decrease chances of conception. (Domar and Kelly, 2002, p. 271)

The following techniques may be useful:

- *Apposition Of Opposites*: for finding a work-life balance.

- *Parts Work*: to resolve inner conflict between the part that wants to get pregnant and the part that wants to continue the unhealthy behaviour, e.g. smoking.

- *Self-Integration Dissociation*: to clear out old unhealthy habits, attitudes and behaviours and bring in a healthy balanced lifestyle.

- *Doors Of Perception*: to experience the effects of an unhealthy attitude vs a healthy attitude on their lifestyle.

- *Mental Rehearsal*: to see themselves having made the changes that they want to make, and experience the positive effects of these changes.

- Direct suggestion: can be useful to help instil new habits.

## Emotional states

### Stress

Stress is a state of tension that occurs when there are too many demands in the environment or when we experience or anticipate experiencing a situation that is perceived as threatening, unpleasant or unfamiliar. As well as having a physical effect on our body, stress can also affect our thoughts, feelings and behaviours (Nejad and Volny, 2008, p. 8). Stress that is too intense, too frequent and/or long lasting is unhealthy and will have a wide range of negative consequences.

Many clients are aware that feeling stressed and anxious is unlikely to help their situation and yet they struggle because they don't know how to go about reducing stress. One client, after at least two years of trying to conceive, told me that she was going to 'throttle the next person' who told her that she just needed to 'relax and it would happen'. Fortunately for me, I had no intention of making that suggestion. Instead I gave her practical and useful advice on how to go about reducing stress which helped her to take control of how she had been feeling.

With fertility problems there are many different factors that may contribute to stress.

Some possible factors include:

- Feeling helpless and out of control
- Having no control over the outcome of treatment
- Monthly disappointment of a menstrual period
- Constant reminders (pregnant women, friends getting pregnant, etc.)
- Feeling unable to achieve a life goal
- Physical stress as a result of tests and treatments
- Financial stress
- Hormonal disruptions
- Personal relationships affected

- Family pressures
- Juggling work and fertility treatments
- Timing sexual intercourse
- Responsibility of decision making
- Waiting for results
- Low success rates for assisted reproductive technology (ART)
- Dealing with treatment failure
- Age and the feeling that time is running out.

*The effect of stress on fertility*

Since stress causes tremendous changes in the body's biochemistry and rhythms it can upset the body's natural balance and over time can lead to chronic health problems. Along with impacting overall health, stress or anxiety over a prolonged period of time can disrupt the production of the hormones needed for ovulation, implantation and sperm quality. Since the body's priority is to keep us out of danger when we are experiencing a threat or stress, taking care of a foetus would only put us under unnecessary strain.

- The hypothalamus regulates both the stress response as well as the sex hormones, which is why excessive stress can lead to anovulation, irregular menstrual cycles, and in more severe cases, to complete suppression of the menstrual cycle.

- Adrenaline is released by the adrenals when we're stressed. Adrenaline helps us escape from danger but it also inhibits the production of progesterone, which is essential for building and maintaining a lining of the uterus, thus impeding fertility.

- Prolactin (usually released by the pituitary gland to stimulate lactation in preparation for nursing) inhibits a woman's fertility so she'll be less likely to conceive during breast feeding. During times of stress, the pituitary emits high levels of prolactin.

- After prolonged stress the sympathetic nervous system can become hyper-stimulated. A hyper-stimulated nervous system sends *less* blood to the uterus and ovaries, thereby impairing their optimal functioning. (Lewis, 2004).

*Steps for decreasing stress*

1. Relaxation techniques need to be used and also taught to the client. An explanation of the following techniques can be found in Section C (Page 181).

    Hypnotic techniques for relaxation:
    - *Progressive relaxation*
    - *Breathing Colour*
    - *Favourite Place / Safe Place*
    - *Resource Gathering*
    - *Hypothalamus Meditation.*

    Self-help tools for relaxation:
    - *7:11 Breathing*
    - *Self-Hypnosis*
    - *Mini-Break Anchor*
    - *Mindfulness*
    - *Quick Body Scan*
    - *Nurturing.*

2. Beliefs that are maintaining the stress need to be challenged.
    For more information please refer to the section on working with beliefs (Page 59).

3. The necessary changes needed in day-to-day life that will help reduce stress.

    Recommendations for reducing stress:
    - Reduce the external stressors that you are able to control
    - Avoid the people who you feel stressed around
    - Reduce the number of activities you are doing that make demands on you
    - Reduce caffeine, alcohol and cigarettes
    - Increase exercise and physical movement
    - Eat small amounts regularly and eat slowly
    - Go to bed early
    - Include relaxation time every day
    - Do *Self-Hypnosis* twice a day

- Take part in activities that you enjoy.

Trying to make all of these changes at once may in itself be stressful. I would recommend small progressive changes to reduce stress, and suggest that *Self-Hypnosis* for relaxation is a priority.

*Depression*

The pioneering work of Dr Alice Domar, founder and executive director of the Domar Center for Complementary Healthcare in Waltham, Massachusetts, has clearly documented that women who've been diagnosed as infertile are twice as likely to be depressed as a control group, and that this depression peaks about two years after they start trying to get pregnant. And even though infertility is not life-threatening, infertile women have depression scores that are indistinguishable from those of women with cancer, heart disease, or HIV (Domar, 1992).

Depression is experienced as a low mood, increasing preoccupation with negative ideas about life and the world, a lack of motivation to do the things you used to enjoy doing, finding things an effort and sleeping poorly.

For some people depression is driven by guilt, for others it may be driven by anxiety or anger. In some cases it may be driven by a combination of all three.

'Major' depression (American Psychiatric Association, 2000) is diagnosed if someone has been experiencing a depressed mood or loss of pleasure in their usual activities, along with four of the following symptoms for at least two weeks:

- Depressed mood
- Loss of pleasure or interest in usual activities
- Disturbance in appetite
- Sleep disturbance
- Feeling agitated or lethargic
- Loss of energy
- Feelings of worthlessness or guilt

- Difficulties in thinking

- Recurrent thoughts of death or suicide.

Research evidence shows that in the vast majority of cases, the depression will lift if treated by effective psychological methods, and that people helped by these methods relapse far less than people given drug treatments (Griffin and Tyrrell, 2004, p. 9).

*The effects of depression on fertility*

Depression can destabilise healthy hormonal balance in the body and negatively affect fertility. One study suggested that depression is associated with abnormal regulation of luteinising hormone (LH), which plays a major role in conception. The immune system is also weakened by depression, which in turn will affect fertility. We also know that if a woman is clinically depressed, she is unable to care for herself, let alone a baby. Infertility may be nature's way of postponing pregnancy until the mother is psychologically capable of raising a child. In the same way that animals in hopeless situations also become less fertile (Domar and Kelly, 2002, p. 30). A study in Germany showed that men in a hopeless situation, namely death row, all had a very low sperm count (Domar and Kelly, 2002).

Women suffering from depression, stress and anxiety are twice as likely to have problems conceiving. In one study 60% of women who were treated for depression got pregnant within a six month period, as opposed to only 24% of untreated women (Nicholas, 2006, p. 49). Another study showed that women who had experienced at least one unsuccessful IVF cycle and who had depressive symptoms before continuing IVF treatment experienced a 13% subsequent pregnancy rate, in contrast to a 29% pregnancy rate in women who did not experience depressive symptoms before their IVF cycle (Domar and Kelly, 2002, p. 24).

*Steps to help lift depression*

Only therapists qualified to do so should work with depression. It may be necessary to refer your client on to a suitable therapist to address the depression before continuing with the next stage of treatment. Below are some suggestions informed by the Human Givens Approach (Griffin and Tyrrell, 2004) which can help lift depression.

1. Relaxation techniques need to be used and also taught to the client.

   Although depressed people may not feel as if they are in a highly aroused state, they do have a high level of stress hormones in their system.

   Depression keeps you locked in your emotional brain and your capacity to think clearly is diminished. Relaxation techniques return a sense of perspective that will help the person deal with the depression more easily.

   Hypnotic techniques for relaxation:
   - *Progressive relaxation*: avoid suggestions of heaviness as people often associate depression with a feeling of heaviness
   - *Breathing Colour:* breathing in a colour which is uplifting and calming
   - *Favourite Place*
   - *Hypothalamus Meditation.*

   Self-help tools for relaxation:
   - *7:11 Breathing*
   - *Self-Hypnosis*
   - *Mini-Break Anchor*
   - *Mindfulness*
   - *Quick Body Scan.*

2. Determine which emotional needs are not being met.

   The following questions form part of the Human Givens full Emotional Needs Audit (ENA) and may help determine which emotional needs are not being met.

   - Do you feel safe?
   - Do you have people in your life who are important to you, and to whom you are important?
   - Do you have wider connections?
   - Are you comfortable with your status in society?
   - Do you have a sense of competence and achievement?
   - Do you have a sense of autonomy and control?
   - Are you receiving and giving attention in a healthy way?
   - Are you being 'stretched' by how you live or the work you do?

For a detailed description of the basic emotional needs and the full Emotional Needs Audit, please refer to the Human Givens Approach (Griffin and Tyrrell, 2004a, p. 90).

3. Set small achievable goals.

   - Goals can be focused on fulfilling unmet needs that may have been identified and on increasing the client's engagement with life.

   - Achieving small goals can help motivate and build confidence to achieve bigger goals.

   - Create a scale for goals to help monitor and identify the changes that have happened between sessions.

   - Scales can also be used to identify the client's resources which have helped bring about those changes. Refer to *Working with scales* for more information (Page 35).

   - The client can create their own scales in a journal to monitor how they feel when they have taken steps towards their goals.

4. Stop worry and negative thinking patterns.
   (Use the methods outlined in the beliefs section and in the section on worry, Page 78.)

5. Develop resources.

   - Use solution focused questions and scaling (Page 35) to continue to identify and develop the client's inner resources.

   - Metaphor and storytelling are effective ways of reminding the client about the resources that they have and how they can be useful in their current situation.

   - Resource gathering: to recall and access skills and resources from past experiences.

6. Positive Mental Rehearsal.

   - Pseudo-orientation techniques can be used to help clients to change their expectation of themselves and their life and to rehearse new behaviours.

*Anxiety*

Anxiety is present when the normal healthy fight-or-flight response is being triggered at unnecessary and inappropriate times. At times this can escalate to a full-blown panic attack. When anxiety is present, balance needs to be restored to the autonomic nervous system.

The short-term consequences of anxiety include dizziness, nausea, shaking, and having scary or negative thoughts. Over prolonged and intense periods of anxiety one's mental, emotional and physical health will be adversely affected.

*Steps to help overcome anxiety*

1. Relaxation techniques can be used in the session and also taught to the client.

    Hypnotic techniques for relaxation:
    - *Progressive relaxation*
    - *Breathing Colour*
    - *Favourite Place*
    - *Resource Gathering*
    - *Hypothalamus Meditation.*

    Self-help tools for relaxation:
    - *7:11 Breathing*
    - *Self-Hypnosis*
    - *Mini-Break Anchor*
    - *Quick Body Scan*
    - *Mindfulness.*

2. Create an external focus of attention.

    Anxiety is kept alive by negative thinking and worry; it is often accompanied by excessive internal focus of attention. Help the client focus outwards and to really look at what is around them. A useful way for them to practise this would be with the self-help tool *Mindfulness*.

3. Dissociate the anxiety.

    Help the client to separate themselves from their anxiety. Anxiety is not an intrinsic part of them but rather an experience they are having.

    This can be done by adapting the *Primal Image* technique, as outlined below.

- *Become aware of the anxiety as a form or a symbol or an image, such as a dark heavy cloud.*
- *Imagine it floating out of you so that you can see it 'over there'.*
- *Become aware of how you can disable it or dissolve it at will, e.g. I can blow it away.*

4. Become aware of negative thoughts.

   - *At times when you feel anxious become aware of what you are thinking.*
   - *Carry a notebook and write down the negative thoughts that you become aware of. This is a useful way to become aware of the thoughts which are fuelling your anxiety.*
   - *Set aside half an hour every day dedicated to worrying. Whenever a worry comes to mind at another time of day, put it aside until it is time to worry.*

5. Modify thinking patterns and challenge negative thoughts.
   (Use the methods outlined in the beliefs section, below.)

6. Teach your client how to find a healthy affirmation.

   - *When you become aware of a repetitive negative thought ask yourself: What you would you prefer to be thinking instead?*
   - *Use this information to create a sentence which is in the present tense and phrased positively, e.g. I can handle this situation in a calm way.*

7. Practise and reinforce the *Affirmation*.

   An affirmation can be used as an effective self-help tool to reinforce and maintain change.

   (Refer to the self-help tools in Section C for a detailed description of *Affirmations*, Page 283.)

## Beliefs

*A recent study at Harvard Medical School measured what happened when women who were having difficulty conceiving were given group CBT. They were taught how to identify recurrent negative thought patterns and how to separate truth from fear. 55% of the women who participated had a baby, compared to 20% who received no treatment.*

(Nicholas, 2006)

Creating mental peace and balance may include addressing the following areas:

- Unhealthy beliefs
- Negative self-talk
- Worry
- Unresolved issues.

Going through problems conceiving and being diagnosed with infertility seems to strongly affect the areas of self-belief, self-worth and hope about life as a whole. Through questions and trance work we can help the client become aware of these resistances and unhealthy beliefs.

To establish mental balance and harmony we need to address any conscious or unconscious resistance to having a baby. Since unconscious blocks are often related to unresolved issues, I have included more information about working with this in *Stage 3: Resolve*. The unhealthy beliefs that may have developed as a result of past experiences and difficulties can be addressed directly as suggested below. When unhealthy beliefs have been identified and challenged, it may be helpful to work to resolve the initiating event in *Stage 3: Resolve*.

*Working with unhealthy beliefs*

The first step in working with an unhealthy belief is to help the client become conscious of it. Firstly, ask the client how they have been feeling. Once an unhealthy emotional state has been identified this way then ask questions to elicit the inderlying belief. Examples of these questions are given below.

Questions that help elicit unhealthy beliefs:

- What is it about this situation that disturbs you the most?
- And what would be so bad about that?
- How do you feel about yourself as a result of the situation you find yourself in?
- If you were to never have children, how would you feel about yourself?

For example, the client may tell you that she has been feeling really jealous lately. She recalls hearing news that a friend of hers had become pregnant with her third child. When she thought about it she recognised that she was most upset by the fact that it just did not seem fair. She had concluded that she obviously didn't deserve to have a child as much as her friend did.

In this example the limiting/unhealthy belief is 'I don't deserve to have a baby'.

The process of *Cognitive Restructuring* can help your client challenge this belief. This process can be taught to the client so that she can do it on her own in between sessions.

*Cognitive Restructuring: challenge an unhealthy belief*

- Does this thought contribute to your _____ (emotional disturbance)?
- Where did you learn this thought?
- Is this thought logical?
- Is this thought true, is it a fact?
- If you were feeling more _____ (healthy emotion) what would you be thinking then?

    Or

- What would you prefer to be thinking that you know would help you to feel better?

The healthy thought that has been identified then needs to be worked with using some of the techniques below in order for it to become integrated as a belief.

*Useful techniques*

- *Doors Of Perception*: increase understanding of the effect of an unhealthy belief, instil a new belief and learn how to come to terms with alternative future possibilities.
- *Apposition Of Opposites*: to create balance in thinking.

- *Anchor*: anchor a healthy emotional state which the client can then access while thinking the healthy thought.

- *Parts Work*: to identify the part responsible for the unhealthy belief, and to access the part responsible for the new healthy belief. Use negotiation to help create inner change.

- EMDR: to desensitise unhealthy belief and install healthy belief.

- EFT: to clear unhealthy belief.

*Homework*

- Find evidence to support the new belief.

- *Cognitive Restructuring*: for any emotional disturbance such as jealousy, anxiety or depression.

- *Affirmations*: to practise and reinforce the new healthy belief. Combine with an anchored resource state.

- *The Orange Dot*: as a cue to trigger healthy affirmation.

*Self-talk*

Negative self-talk and worry fuel anxiety. Often clients are not consciously aware of their inner dialogue and fail to realise the effect that their thinking is having on them. Creating mental wellbeing will often mean that the client needs to become more aware of their own inner dialogue.

As young children, we are directed and disciplined by adults who tell us that we 'must/have to/should/ought to ... ' do this or that. Words such as these are very effective ways of imposing rules and demands. As adults, many of us have internalised these voices, and continue to talk to ourselves using these stress words. When we use these words in our self-talk we are implying that we have no choice in the matter, which leads to feelings of pressure and stress. For example: 'I really *should* clean the house.' or 'I really *ought to* do more *Self-Hypnosis*.' Eradicating these stress words can make you feel empowered and free to choose what it is you will or won't do. Stress words can be replaced by words that imply choice and flexibility rather than demands and pressure. For example: 'I would *prefer* to clean the house,' or 'I *could* do more *Self-Hypnosis*.'

Steps to create healthy self-talk:

1. Suggest that the client carries a journal and writes down any negative thoughts they become aware of and makes note of the times when they are using stress words such as: must, have to, should, ought to.

2. Challenge the negative self-talk using the *Cognitive Restructuring* exercise.

3. Make a note of a new way of thinking about it.

4. Replace stress words with words that indicate preference and choice.

5. Teach *Self-Talk SUDS* as a self-help tool.

*Worry*

Worrying may be a way of life for some people, and others find that their fertility problems have resulted in them worrying more. Worry is a form of negative self-hypnosis and a misguided use of the imagination. I often have clients tell me that they seem to worry a lot about things related to their fertility and that they recognise that worrying is negatively affecting how they feel.

Often people worry about things because they somehow think that worrying is going to either prevent something 'bad' happening or help the situation in some way. Assisting your clients in recognising that worrying isn't in fact helpful can empower them to use their imagination in a way that can positively affect their situation.

Below are a few simple steps to suggest to clients to help them *Worry Less:*

1. Pay attention and notice when you are worrying.

2. Ask yourself, 'Is there anything I can do about this now?' If there is something that can be done, do it.

3. If nothing can be done, ask yourself, 'Is worrying about this helping me now?' If not, you can then choose to stop worrying.

4. If you continue to notice yourself worrying, set aside a 'worry half-hour' every day. If you catch yourself worrying outside of this time, make a

note of what you are worrying about and then wait until the designated time to worry.

5. When you notice worrying and intrusive thoughts, mentally say 'STOP'.

*Modifying thought patterns*

The following scripts can be used, whilst the client is in trance, for interrupting negative self-talk or worry.

*Become aware of some of the things that you worry about …*

*Take a moment to just let yourself start to worry about one of those things. (Pause) In a few moments I will ask you to STOP that worry by imagining a big red STOP sign, and hearing yourself say the word 'STOP' very clearly and loudly in your mind. As soon as you see that STOP sign and hear yourself say the word 'STOP', immediately that worry can stop, and you will be able to think about something more useful, something more pleasant, something that helps you feel better. For now, just let yourself worry. (Pause) Now STOP. Imagine that red STOP sign and hear your own inner voice saying 'STOP'. Now allow yourself to think about something you would prefer to think about.* (Repeat this paragraph three times.)

*Now, whenever you notice worrying thoughts, you can immediately see that red STOP sign and hear the word 'STOP', and as soon as you do, that worrying will STOP and you will be free to think about something that helps you feel better …*

*The two week wait*

The two weeks spent waiting for pregnancy results after IVF implantation is often a very difficult time for women. Teaching them tools for interrupting worry and challenging negative self-talk can be very helpful for them at this time. To find out more about working with clients during the two week wait, please see *The 4 Session Plan For IVF* (Page 332).

# *Physical symptoms and hormonal balance*

Physical symptoms including Polycystic Ovarian Syndrome, endometriosis, low sperm count, poor sperm mobility and hormonal imbalances (high follicle stimulating hormone levels, low testosterone and so on) can be improved through emotional balance and positive lifestyle changes. Mind-body approaches can also be used to investigate specific emotional factors that may be affecting the condition or visualisation techniques can be used to create physiological changes. More information about how to use mind-body techniques to restore physical wellbeing and enhance fertility can be found in *Stage 4: Enhance* (Page 125). Many of the ideas and techniques mentioned in Stage 3 will be useful for resolving past events which are causing or affecting current physical conditions. There is also a discussion about how to restore menstrual health in *Stage 3: Resolve* (Page 89).

Some of the common physical symptoms that may need to be addressed include:

- Endometriosis
- Polycystic Ovarian Syndrome (PCOS)
- Irregular cycles and anovulation
- Menstrual health problems
- Low sperm count
- Poor sperm motility
- Other hormonal imbalances such as oestradiol, progesterone, luteinising hormone or testosterone
- High follicle stimulating hormone (FSH) levels.

*Useful techniques*

- *Primal Image*: can be adapted and used to help restore wellbeing to any physical condition. Access a primal image for the relevant organ or body system.

- *Control Room*: to adjust the controls for the relevant systems and/or organs of the body. When working with high hormone levels such as high FSH, visualise the dial for FSH being turned down to a healthy level.

- *Apposition Of Opposites*: a very effective mind-body technique for encouraging hormonal balance. Use it to restore balance to the menstrual cycle.

- *Healing White Light*: to cleanse and clear the body of anything that may be negatively affecting physical wellbeing.

- *Inner Guide*: to access unconscious wisdom and guidance about how to restore wellbeing.

- *Parts Work*: to identify the part responsible for a particular condition, to elicit the positive intention and purpose of the part responsible.

- *Connect With Your Inner Body*: to create hormonal balance and restore regular rhythm to the body.

- *Body Talk*: to determine if any emotional factors are affecting physical problems. To ask the body what it needs for health to be restored.

- *Hypothalamus Meditation*: to reduce the effects of stress on the reproductive system and create hormonal balance.

- *The Big Race*: to improve sperm motility.

## Case study: high FSH levels

High FSH levels are often of concern to the clients that I see, but I have found that mind-body approaches can have a good effect on balancing these hormone levels.

FSH levels are often tested to determine how much effort is being expended by a woman's body to produce viable eggs for reproductive purposes. If a woman is not producing quality follicles, her FSH levels increase in an effort to correct the situation (Schwartz, 2008, p. 59). If FSH levels are higher than 10 it can indicate that there is a reduced number of viable eggs left in the ovaries. However, many women with high FSH levels have normal fertility. High levels may be a problem for stimulation treatment which requires the body to produce multiple eggs in a single cycle (Lockwood et al, S, 2007).

Jillian, aged 38, came to see me after it had been confirmed that her FSH levels were 22. She had done a few months of repeat testing but the results seemed to be fairly conclusive.

As a result, one of her main aims for coming to see me was to reduce her FSH levels. Jillian and her husband had been trying to conceive for about a year, and aside from her FSH test results there seemed to be no other problems with either of them.

Her demanding job as a TV producer meant that she often worked very long hours for long periods of time. This, coupled with her growing concern about her fertility, left her feeling very stressed.

Once we had created a clear goal for therapy, I singled out one of her top priorities, which was to reduce stress. Using solution focused questions I asked Jillian to tell me more about what it would be like when she had reduced her feelings of stress. I then got her to rate herself on a scale now, where 10 represented her living and experiencing these reduced levels of stress. She felt that she was currently at a 2.

Most of our first session together was spent on the goal setting, case history and education. I explained to her that the hypothalamus is a small gland located at the base of the brain which communicates with the pituitary gland to control the flow of hormones in the body and that stress can affect the functioning of the hypothalamus and cause a disruption to hormonal balance, including FSH levels.

During the first consultation we also did a short session of deep relaxation together using the *Safe Place* script. In trance I taught her how she could access this deep relaxation on her own and suggested that she could practise this for ten minutes twice a day. Along with her twice daily relaxation I suggested that she also make a long list of the things that she found relaxing and enjoyed doing.

In the second session a week later Jillian told me that she was now a 4 on the scale. She'd been doing her relaxation every day and had become much more conscious of her stress levels which meant that she had started doing more things to help herself feel better. I asked her to tell me more about the things she had been doing and then got her to identify ways in which she could continue doing more of the same. She also brought along her list of relaxing activities and we looked at how she could incorporate one or two of them into the week ahead. I taught her about the *Emotional Bank Account* and asked her to pay close attention to her Emotional Bank Account over the coming weeks. After some deep relaxation I used the *Free Floating Pseudo-orientation* to take her to a time in the future in which she had realised her goal, was feeling calmer and her FSH levels were in balance. This technique served the dual purpose of allowing her to experience her goal state and all the benefits and effects, as well as being a resource gathering tool which allowed her to bring back resources and learning from the future time.

The following week, having continued on with daily relaxation and using the *Emotional Bank Account* to keep track of her 'incomings' and 'outgoings', Jillian said she was 'at least an 8' on the scale. Once again I began the trance work with the same deep relaxation and then asked her to follow a path into the *Control Room* of her body where she located the dial for her FSH levels. I asked her to notice the current settings, and notice where a healthy balanced setting would be. I suggested that she follow her instincts and make the needed changes to the controls of her reproductive system, and specifically ensure that the FSH levels dial is turned to its optimum setting. I suggested that she could visit her *Control Room* regularly to make any necessary adjustments so that noticeable changes could happen in the months ahead.

A month later when I saw Jillian again, she looked like a different person. She had made some significant changes to her work life and had continued practising her relaxation and *Control Room* visualisation regularly. I then worked with the *Primal Image* to generate a positive healthy picture of her ovaries and womb and did some *Future Pacing* so that she could see and imagine the positive effects that these changes would have on her life. Jillian grinned from ear to ear during the trance and told me that she could see herself heavily pregnant.

> A month later she rang to tell me that her most recent FSH test was 14, a significant decrease. Although it was not yet within the healthy range, she felt sure that given enough time and self-care it would be.

This case study is one of many anecdotes about women whose FSH levels have gone down or normalised during treatment with me. Sometimes it is necessary to work with more complex underlying issues which may be contributing to stress, but often a very simple, direct approach addressing lifestyle factors and increasing relaxation can make a significant difference.

## Relationship issues

Problems having children can create great strain and stress on a relationship. In some cases, relationship counselling may be helpful. If you are working individually with partners and relationship issues come up, it may be necessary to refer one of the partners on to another therapist in order to work effectively and maintain client confidentiality.

If a couple has been trying to conceive for a long time, their sexual relationship may have become pressurised and mechanical. Trying to have 'sex on demand' at specific times for the sole purpose of getting pregnant will inevitably lead to a lack of intimacy and pleasure.

Suggest that they think about being intimate with each other, without having intercourse, or that they also make love on the woman's infertile days, so that sex can be about more than just having a baby.

When couples have made lots of lifestyle changes to try and improve their fertility or when they have been going through medical treatments for a long time, they sometimes find that they spend less time together doing the things that they enjoy doing.

To restore balance to a relationship the following questions may be helpful:

- What do the two of you enjoy doing together?
- What would you like to do more of?
- What do you know would be good for you both right now?

- Tell me about some of the good times you have had together?

- What would increase spontaneity and pleasure in your sexual relationship?

- What conditions would you need to create so that the two of you could really enjoy making love again?

- What were you like when you first got together?

- What could you do to return a sense of spontaneity to your relationship?

*Approaches*

- *Anchor*: anchor a positive past time in their relationship.

- *Mental Rehearsal*: to see themselves being more spontaneous, playful, etc., and enjoying being with each other.

- *Breathing Colour*: relaxation to reduce stress and pressure so that sex can be more enjoyable.

- *Regression*: to access resources of positive past experiences in their relationship.

## Spiritual beliefs

Your client's spiritual beliefs can be a wonderful resource to work with therapeutically. When people are experiencing emotional turmoil they're likely to want to withdraw and disconnect socially. Many people find that their spirituality is a means of helping them re-establish their sense of connection with life. Working on a spiritual level can remind people that they are bigger than their problem. A belief in a divine plan can help some people to feel a deeper sense of acceptance for what is happening, which in itself can ease a lot of suffering.

The following questions may help identify your client's spiritual resources:

- Have you ever had religious beliefs or spiritual practices?

- Have those been helpful in any way?

- Is there any religious or spiritual figure or activity that you think would be helpful for you in this situation?

- Is there any area of your inner or spiritual life that you would like to develop more?

Spiritual beliefs can also contribute to unhealthy emotions, as is the case when clients believe that God is punishing them for something that they have done in the past. Religious beliefs can also impact on a couple's choice to have fertility treatment. According to some religions, treatments such as IVF go against God's will. Some couples choose to 'secretly' go ahead with treatment because they are aware that their family and community may not agree. This may leave them feeling guilty or conflicted in some way. Working to resolve these conflicts may be necessary in order to maximise their chances of conceiving. More information about working with inner conflicts can be found in *Stage 3: Resolve* (Page 98).

## *Inner resources*

Identifying and developing the client's inner resources is an essential part of the *Fertile Body Method* and should be included in every treatment plan in one form or another.

Typically a 'resource' is anything that will help a person reach a desired state or transform a problem state (Dilts and De Lozier, 2000). Inner resources may come in the form of behaviours or actions, inner states, capabilities, skills or tools, empowering beliefs or spiritual values. Resources can be accessed from personal history, by modelling others or by acting as if something is already true.

We know that faced with a difficult situation or decision everyone will respond differently. The difference in response to difficult situations is often connected to our perception of our own coping abilities.

> *This perception of yourself is based on your personal emotional history. It may be due to past childhood influences and conditioning, beliefs, religion, or your social environment, but it is your perception of your inability to cope that causes the stress response in your body, rather than any external factor.*
>
> (Shapiro, 2008, p. 23)

A key task in *Stage 2: Balance* is to help clients identify and attend to their skills, abilities and resources. This process not only constructs a narrative of the client as a competent individual, but also helps them identify new ways of bringing these resources to bear upon the problem. Identifying the client's strengths and resources builds their own belief in their ability to cope.

A combination of solution focused approaches and hypnotic techniques can help the client to access and develop the skills and resources needed to reach the goal, to deal with the problem in a better way, and to address any difficult or traumatic issues that need to be resolved.

*Approaches*

Solution focused approaches can help identify and develop strengths and resources in the following ways:

- Problem-free talk: ask them how they spend their time and what things they enjoy or have enjoyed in the past.

- Exception-seeking: there are always times when the problem is less severe or absent, so encourage the client to describe what different circumstances existed, or what the client did differently:
  - *Tell me about the times (the problem) does not happen?*
  - *What were you doing differently during these times?*
  - *Tell me about the times that bits of what you want already occur?*
  - *What (belief, ability, state or behaviour) would make it impossible for (the problem) to continue?*

- Find out how they have coped: be curious about how they cope, how they manage to hang on despite adversity. Coping questions are designed to elicit information about client resources that will have gone unnoticed by them. This can be especially important for those who have experienced a lot of difficulties and have been struggling with fertility problems for years. Even the most hopeless story has within it examples of coping that can be drawn out:
  - *I can see that things have been really difficult for you, yet I am struck by the fact that, even so, you manage to get up each morning and do everything necessary to get yourself off to work. How do you do that?*

- Past success: find out what they are already doing or have done in the past that might contribute to their goal being realised:
  - *Have you ever been able to resolve or overcome a problem such as this before? What did you do?*
  - *How did you do that?*
  - *How did you know to do that?*
  - *How did you know that doing that would be good for you?*
  - *What difference did that make?*
  - *In what way was that good for you?*

- *Who noticed?*
- *How did s/he show you that s/he had noticed?*
- *How did that show?*
- *What did it take?*
- *What does doing that tell you about yourself?*
- *If things had gone better how would (could) you have known?*

- External resources: ask questions that will help them learn from and model other peoples successes:
  - *Do you know anyone who has managed to overcome (this problem)? What did they do?*

- Scaling questions: in follow-up sessions scales created in the first session can be revisited and used to help identify resources:
  - *Where are you on the scale now? (If they are up on the scale) How did you do that?*
  - *(If they are down on the scale) What's stopping you from slipping one point lower down the scale?*
  - *On days when you are one point higher on the scale, what are you doing differently? How do you do that?*
  - *If you did have the resources you need in order to reach your goal, what would they be?*
  - *If you were already a 10 on the scale, and you were looking back, what would you see that you had done in order to accomplish that?*

Hypnotic approaches to develop and build resources include:

- *Resource Gathering*
- *Regression*
- *Parts Work*
- *Safe Place*
- *Anchors*
- *Inner Guide*
- *Self-Integration Dissociation*
- *Free Floating Pseudo-orientation*
- *Mental Rehearsal*
- Storytelling/Metaphor.

## *Stage 3: Resolve*

Stage 3 of the *Fertile Body Method* addresses the issues that your client may need to resolve to achieve their goal and move them towards their intention of having a child. Personally, I find this stage of treatment incredibly fascinating. There is still so much about fertility that medical experts don't understand, and I think the area of unresolved issues provides yet another piece to this complex puzzle. While science has given some explanations about how unresolved issues may affect fertility, it is always interesting for me to hear what clients consciously or unconsciously feel is affecting their fertility. In my experience of working with fertility clients it certainly seems that resolving these issues often results in parenthood. I have yet to do my own statistical research into this, but I do know that other therapists have found as much as a 45% success rate when addressing underlying and unresolved issues (Greaves, 2002).

Identifying which issues need to be resolved is the key to working successfully in this stage of treatment. We are all in a constant state of growing, changing and healing and at any given time there may be a number of issues that need to be resolved. This stage in the *Fertile Body Method* is specifically for addressing those things that are related to the client's goal. Bearing this in mind will help you keep your sessions focused and relevant. It is important, however, not to limit this stage of treatment to resolving issues that *you* think are related to the goal.

In this section I have included some ideas about how you and your client can identify what the issues are that may need to be addressed. There are of course clients for whom this stage of treatment is not relevant because there are no unresolved issues that have a bearing on their goal for therapy. In these cases, *Stage 1: Outcome* and *Stage 2: Balance* may be followed by *Stage 4: Enhance* or *Stage 5: Prepare*.

In order to put this work in context I have included some thoughts about why resolution is important for fertility. In this book I am merely touching on these ideas and encourage you to further investigate this fascinating area of the mind-body relationship.

Experienced therapists are likely to have a whole host of ways of working with unresolved issues. For those newer to the field, I have included an overview of some of the approaches that I use in this stage of the *Fertile Body Method*. I have also included a more detailed discussion about the following areas that often come up in my work: unconscious blocks (which include a general approach for working with unresolved issues), age, previous terminations, miscarriage, stillbirth and neonatal death, trauma, menstrual health, and parenthood.

I strongly recommend that you work through *Stage 1: Outcome* and *Stage 2: Balance* of the Method before addressing any unresolved issues. Not only is this a safe way of working, but I have had numerous cases who have 'spontaneously' resolved issues once they have a clear goal and access to their inner resources.

---

### Case study: indirectly resolving issues

The following case is a good illustration of how something can be resolved without needing to work directly with it.

When Dana came to see me she said that she knew that the guilt she was feeling about having terminated a pregnancy was getting in the way of conceiving. When I asked her how she knew this she told me that she had been having a recurring dream over the past few months during which she was giving birth. She dreamt that instead of giving birth to a baby, she delivered an aborted foetus. She would wake up from this dream feeling heavy with guilt. Part of her goal for treatment was to resolve this issue and feel at peace with herself.

In the first session we spent some time gathering specific information about what that resolution would be like for her and how she would know when this issue had been resolved. I used the solution focused scales to help her identify where she was in relation to her goal now and what small changes she would notice when she began moving up that scale. In the *Stage 2: Balance*, we worked with the *Self-Integration Dissociation* to mobilise her inner resources and wisdom. During the *Self-Integration Dissociation* I asked her to use her in-breath to breathe in the resources that she needed in order to resolve this issue.

She told me at her next session two weeks later that she had dreamt that she was wandering around inside her boundary and had found a magical mirror. She had sat down in front of the mirror where she could see her own reflection staring back at her. Her reflection told her that this was a forgiveness mirror and that anything that was revealed to this mirror could be forgiven. She looked into her own eyes which looked back at her with compassion and told the mirror about her termination. She cried as she told the mirror all about that time in her life and why she had done what she did. When she was finished, she saw her reflection looking back lovingly at her as it told her that all had been forgiven. When she awoke from this dream she felt as if she had shed a weight and told me that she now knew she was at a 10 on the solution focused scale that we had created. I found her experience so touching and inspiring that I went on to develop it into a visualisation which I call *The Mirror Of Forgiveness* (Page 272).

In cases where the issues that need to be resolved are not conscious or when this kind of 'spontaneous' resolution does not happen, the information, techniques and approaches in this section will be helpful. When it is necessary to work directly with unresolved issues in order to enhance fertility, I would remind you only to do so if you are fully qualified and equipped in this area. This is particularly important where there has been sexual or physical abuse and/or severe trauma.

**This section contains:**
- The importance of resolution for fertility
- Who is to blame?
- How to identify issues that may need to be resolved
- Some possible approaches for resolution
- Some possible issues to resolve
- Some possible areas of inner conflict
  - Unconscious blocks
  - Age
  - Previous terminations
  - Miscarriage
  - Stillbirth and neonatal death
  - Menstrual health
  - Parenthood.

## *The importance of resolution for fertility*

I have heard many people describe their fertility journey as 'a journey to wholeness'. Fertility problems have the potential of taking people down a path of self-reflection and healing. In their quest to conceive they learn to overcome problems and issues that may have been affecting them for many years. While I believe that this in itself is incredibly valuable, I also believe that resolving many of these issues can play a vital role in preparing the body for conception, pregnancy and birth. This is as important for natural conception as it is for those undergoing assisted reproduction.

## The Fertile Body Method

*Unresolved and unexpressed emotional and psychological stress has physiological consequences that may hamper the effectiveness of fertility treatments.*
(Facchinetti et al, 1997)

During the past ten years there has been a growing body of research showing how the mind and body respond to each other, clearly demonstrating how emotional and psychological states translate into altered responses in the chemical balance of the body (Shapiro, 2008).

*All our experiences from conception to now are stored in the emotional brain – some of these experiences we remember, many of them are stored in the subconscious. Emotions such as anger, fear or depression are our responses to these experiences. The brain transforms these emotions into biochemical and electrical messages from the hypothalamus and pituitary glands and they are distributed throughout the body via the bloodstream. This negative hormonal communication along the hypothalamic-pituitary-gonad axis is responsible for many reproductive problems. Research is now showing that resolving unfinished business from childhood and earlier adult life can impact positively on our hormonal systems, thereby enhancing our ability to conceive and birth a healthy baby.*
(Payne, 1997)

Neuropeptides are the chemical messengers that carry information from the mind to the body and vice versa. These neuropeptides which are secreted by the brain, the immune system and nerve cells, can carry information to every cell in the body and influence the behaviour of that cell. Neuropeptides provide the link between thoughts, perceptions and feelings and the physical responses that occur in the cells and systems of the body.

*In other words, you can't have an idea or a notion, or a thought or a feeling, or a desire without your immune cells actually knowing about it. The immune cells are eavesdropping on your internal dialogue, they're literally listening to the conversation that you are having with yourself in every second of your existence.*
(Chopra, 2000)

*When we experience emotions, we experience a biochemical change in our bodies. Emotions exist both as energy and molecules of matter in the receptors of every cell in the body.*
(Pert, 1999)

*What we find is that any emotion that is repressed, denied or ignored will get stuck in the body. As Candace Pert defines it: 'Your body is your subconscious mind.' In other words, the thoughts and emotions you are not acknowledging, dealing with, resolving or healing will simply make themselves known elsewhere.*

(Shapiro, 2008)

Issues that are unresolved in the unconscious mind remain trapped in the body and can affect fertility.

*Thoughts have energy; emotions have energy. They make you do and say things and act in certain ways. They make you jump up and down or lie prone in bed. They determine what you eat and who you love. The energy behind what you think and feel does not just disappear if it is held back or repressed. When you cannot or do not express what is happening on an emotional or psychological level, that feeling becomes embodied (you take it deeper within yourself) until it manifests through the physical body.*

(Shapiro, 2008)

I would consider an issue from the past unresolved if the client recalls the past event and finds that they experience a distressing emotional or physical response to that memory and/or they experience a response when they think about a possible future event which consciously or unconsciously reminds them of something unresolved from the past. These emotional responses to past events are deeply entwined with the beliefs that the client holds about themselves. Unresolved issues will often highlight the underlying negative or limiting beliefs that the clients holds. So in essence, resolution occurs when the emotional response and the limiting belief are no longer accessed in relation to that memory. In Section B, *Stage 2: Balance* I discuss how unhealthy beliefs can affect our physiology (Page 59) and I feel that this is one way of understanding why resolution is important for fertility.

Fortunately, hypnosis is a very effective way of working with unresolved issues and unconscious blocks to conception, pregnancy, birth and parenthood. Dr Elizabeth Muir, a clinical psychologist who specialises in treating fertility problems using counselling and hypnotherapy, believes that addressing psychological issues can significantly increase the chances of conception.

> *"Hypnotherapy works on the premise that the conscious and subconscious minds may be at odds with each other," she says. "I believe that while a woman might consciously want a baby, her subconscious may be stopping her from getting pregnant. Most women I see have psychosomatic infertility related to conflicts or unresolved issues about having a baby. A combination of counselling and hypnotherapy can remove these problems."*
>
> (Greaves, 2002)

There have been many informative books written about the relationship between the mind and body that provide an in-depth, scientific explanation of how unresolved issues can affect the body. If you are not familiar with this topic I encourage you to read some of the books suggested in the recommended reading list (Page 351) to enrich your understanding of the importance of resolution in fertility.

## *Who is to blame?*

There are many clients who come to see me already blaming themselves for their infertility. The more that these clients learn about the mind-body relationship, the more they are left believing that they can't conceive or carry full term because of something they have done. Helping your clients to understand how past events may affect fertility is a means to empower them and show them how they can positively influence their situation, rather than leaving them feeling that it is their fault.

Sometimes it is important to make it explicitly clear to clients that they are not to blame for what is going on as blaming themselves only adds fuel to the fire. It would be blinkered to think that mental and emotional issues are solely responsible for fertility problems, since this would be denying all the many other influencing factors including the magical, mysterious intelligence and timing of nature. While we may be responsible for the sails of our boat, we are not solely responsible for the sailing as the wind and waters have their role to play. If your client does tend to blame herself, it may be worth exploring this belief more deeply using hypnosis. *Parts Work*, *IMR Signals* and *Regression* are techniques that could assist her in gaining the necessary insights and understanding for shifting this unhealthy belief and changing her perspective.

Essentially we are helping clients reach a place of compassion and love for themselves and for all that they have done and experienced. When they are able to accept and forgive themselves for what they did or did not do, then they have a context in which resolution can truly occur. *The Mirror Of Forgiveness* can be used in this way. Alternatively, the boundary in the *Self-Integration Dissociation* can be built with love and kindness so that when they are inside their inner world they are surrounded by love and compassion. This will allow them to look at what or who they blame with kindness and compassion. In one case, a client described to me how she saw her 'old self' who had abused her body with drugs and food simply dissolve and wash away as she looked onto her with the feelings of love emanating from her boundary. Up until then she had held her 'old self' responsible for her fertility problems and had been blaming herself for her 'old eggs'.

If fertility is a journey to wholeness, the acknowledgement and acceptance of all parts of oneself is a fundamental aspect of this work.

## *How to identify issues that may need to be resolved*

The first aspect of this stage is to identify what issues need to be resolved. Sometimes it is blatantly obvious to the therapist and the client what needs to be resolved; at other times you may intuitively feel that there is something underlying that the client is not consciously aware of. Learning how to identify the issues that need to be resolved is an essential step in this stage of treatment. I believe that the client will consciously or unconsciously know what needs to be addressed.

Below are some of the ways that you can identify these issues:

- The client will tell you. For example: 'My relationship with my mother is really getting in the way of believing that I can be a good parent.'

- You hear or see it in the case history. The client may not explicitly mention an issue but you hear that there is something that has not been fully addressed or dealt with. Seeing a change in body language, voice and posture may draw this to your attention.

- Listen to the client's language and make a note of any negative or limiting beliefs the client holds. For example, the client may say, 'I've always known that I would have problems conceiving,' 'It's just typical that something like this would happen to me,' or 'With all of this going on my husband probably wishes he had married someone else'.

- Allow the issues to naturally unfold during the course of therapy. When the client feels safe with the therapist and good rapport has been established, it is more likely that the client will tell you about past traumas and unresolved issues. The work that you do together in *Stage 1: Outcome* and *Stage 2: Balance* may help the client become more aware of what their limiting beliefs and unresolved issues are. Sometimes issues that need to be addressed are brought to the client's awareness spontaneously during a trance session.

- Set homework tasks. Setting the client homework tasks will help them become more conscious of what their fears and limiting beliefs around having a child are. For example, ask them to think about and write down all the reasons why they want to have children and all the reasons why they don't want to have children.

- Premenstrual symptoms. Ask the client to take note of thoughts and feelings that arise prior to menstruation. These symptoms can highlight unresolved issues which may need to be addressed. More information about this can be found in the menstrual health section (Page 115).

- Ask the unconscious mind. There are many different techniques and ways of doing this which I have described in the section titled *Unconscious Blocks* (Page 99).

## *Some possible approaches for resolution*

Once the issues have been identified, the next step is to work with them to bring about resolution. Resolution occurs when the event no longer creates emotional disturbance and the beliefs resulting from the event are no longer limiting or unhealthy. Obtain conscious/unconscious confirmation that this issue is no longer negatively affecting the client's goal.

I have found the following approaches to be effective ways of working with unresolved issues:

- Desensitising visualisation techniques can help resolve phobias and trauma. Examples of these types of techniques are the *Rewind Technique* (also called the Fast Phobia Cure), Hypno-desensitisation and Two stage dissociation. The *Rewind Technique* can be found in Section C (Page 206). These techniques are useful for addressing things such as:
    - Birth trauma
    - Needle phobia
    - Miscarriage
    - Stillbirth

- Termination of pregnancy
- Sexual abuse
- Rape.

- Hypno-analytical techniques give the client insight and understanding so that they can resolve issues around inner conflict. These hypno-analytical techniques include *Parts Work*, *IMR Signals* and *Regression* and can be found in Section C (Page 181).
  Hypno-analytical techniques are particularly good for:
    - Termination of pregnancy
    - Relationship problems
    - Parenthood
    - Sexual performance problems
    - Issues and conflict about career vs family
    - Limiting beliefs.

- *Cognitive Restructuring* to challenge unhealthy beliefs that may have been created as a result of a past event. Past experiences can be resolved by changing the unhealthy belief that is causing the current emotional disturbance into a healthy belief.
    - Previous termination, e.g. 'I don't deserve to have a baby.'
    - Miscarriage, e.g. 'It's my fault that I had a miscarriage.'
    - Parenting, e.g. 'I won't be able to cope with being a mother.'

- Metaphorical approaches to working indirectly with the unresolved issue. These techniques can be done content free and are gentle, non-invasive ways of working with disturbing issues.

- Talking about unresolved past events is sometimes all the client may need to feel that they have reached closure. This seems to be especially true in cases where the client may not have discussed this issue with anyone ever before.

- EMDR (Eye Movement Desensitisation and Reprocessing) is an information processing therapy developed by Francine Shapiro to resolve symptoms relating to disturbing and unresolved life experiences. More information about EMDR can be found in Section E (Page 355).

- EFT (Emotional Freedom Technique) works by tapping acupressure points on the body. This releases emotions connected to unresolved issues. I have found that EFT is a very rapid, effective and direct way of working with unresolved issues. Please refer to Section E for more information on EFT (Page 355).

## Some possible issues to resolve

There are a vast number of possible issues to resolve which may be negatively affecting mental, emotional or physical wellbeing. Generally, any belief or emotional response that is in conflict with the client's goal and/or their desire to have a child may need to be resolved. The following list gives some common examples of past events that may result in blocks to fertility (Schwartz, 2008):

- Any past trauma
- Previous terminations
- Miscarriage
- Stillbirth and neonatal death
- Sexual abuse
- Rape
- Issues with one's own birth and conception
- Dysfunctional family relationships
- Ancestral/ Inherited issues.

## Some possible areas of inner conflict

Psychological factors affecting fertility can be thought of in terms of past events, or current beliefs and inner conflicts. The following list includes some typical examples of inner conflicts that a client with fertility problems may have:

- Fears about pregnancy, birth, hospitals
- Fear of having a deformed/disabled child
- Fear of losing their independence
- Concerns about the effect of having a baby on their relationship
- Career vs family conflict

- Concerns about body image
- Ambivalence about parenthood
- Will my husband be a good father?
- Will my husband leave me?
- Will I cope as a mother?
- Not wanting to repeat their parents' shortcomings
- Believing they must be a perfect mother
- Sexual problems
- Not believing it is possible to have a child.

## *Unconscious blocks*

The examples given above may or may not be in the client's conscious awareness. When I refer to 'blocks' I am referring to the unconscious resistance or internal conflict the client may have in relation to having a baby. When parts of the client are not in alignment with their desire to have a child, it seems to cause internal stress in the mind-body which may directly affect or contribute to fertility problems. Essentially the root of these 'blocks' can be found in unresolved past events and experiences.

Sometimes while talking with the client they will mention that they are aware of a belief that is in conflict with their desire to have a baby. In one case a woman mentioned that her mother had conceived her 'by accident' out of wedlock. As a result she had been brought up being taught 'not to get pregnant by mistake'. Ever since she was a child, she remembers learning that getting pregnant is 'bad' or 'wrong' and that she must 'be careful'. She had developed a belief that 'It is not okay to get pregnant'.

Using *IMR Signals*, her unconscious mind confirmed that this belief was preventing her from conceiving. It was only after we had done some work together (see below) on changing that belief at an unconscious level that she conceived. Rationally she knew that it was not 'wrong and bad' for her to get pregnant, but that belief had been so deeply ingrained in her psyche that her body continued to respond to it until she unconsciously recognised that it was safe and appropriate for her to conceive now.

*Parts Work* helped her communicate with the part responsible for believing that getting pregnant was wrong and unsafe. She thanked the part for looking after her and helping her not get pregnant at times when she really didn't want to have a baby. In trance she explained to the part that it no longer needed to protect her in this way because she was now ready to have a baby and it was now an appropriate thing to do. After communicating with the part in this way she felt the part change from a hot prickly pain in her hand to a warm comforting feeling. She confirmed that the part now knew that it was okay for her to have a baby. *IMR Signals* confirmed that her unconscious mind had taken on this new belief and that she was now free to conceive. Within three months she became pregnant. In cases like this it certainly seems that her old belief was strongly contributing to her inability to conceive. In other cases, unconscious blocks seem to be just one aspect of the problem.

In another example of working with unconscious blocks, a woman told me that she had been very sick as a young teenager. She had been taken to hospital where they discovered that one of her Fallopian tubes had become infected and it was poisoning her whole system. She remembers overhearing her mother talking to the doctors, asking if this would mean that she would never be able to have children. Although the event did not render her infertile, she developed a belief that she would not be able to conceive. Since then she had always told herself and others that she may not be able to have children.

I have also had clients tell me that they feel as if something is blocking them from conceiving. Although they are not consciously aware of what it is, they believe that there may be a past experience that is contributing to the difficulty they have been having. There have also been times when I have intuitively felt that there is something unconscious which may be affecting their fertility.

In both cases, hypnosis can be used to help them recognise if there is a block and/or what the block may be. I don't believe it is always necessary for the client to have conscious awareness of what this block is in order for it to be cleared; hypnosis can be used to create the change on an unconscious level. I normally ask the unconscious mind, using *IMR Signals*, to indicate whether it is safe and appropriate for them to become consciously aware of the block. If it is not, I ask their unconscious mind if this issue can be resolved without them becoming consciously aware of it. Sometimes it is not possible for this unconscious resolution, in which case I would ask the unconscious mind if it would be willing to revisit this issue in the future. I would end this session by asking the unconscious mind to identify what inner resources are needed, if any, in order for the client to be able to resolve this issue at a future time. Some of the ideas and approaches in *Stage 2: Balance* can then be used to mobilise inner resources and build ego strength (Page 62).

If, however, their unconscious mind indicates that it is necessary for them to become conscious of this resistance it is important that the therapist confirms, using *IMR Signals*, that it is safe and appropriate to do so.

## Questions

The following questions will assist the client in identifying any blocks they may have:

- Do you have any fears or concerns about pregnancy, birth or parenthood?
- If there was something mental or emotional affecting your ability to have a baby, what would it be?
- What are some of the reasons you don't want to have a baby?
- What do you feel is holding you back in your life?
- What are some of the thoughts that come to mind when you think about having a baby?

## Direct approaches

The following techniques are useful for working with the unconscious mind to identify blocks, gain insight and negotiate change:

- *IMR Signals:* to locate past events.
- *Parts Work:* to identify inner conflicts.
- *Somatic Bridge Regression*: can be used to identify the root cause of a feeling which is related to fertility, such as failure or guilt.
- *Free Floating Regression*: to identify a past event that may be impacting on the current situation.

- *Cellular Memory Recall*: to get insight into any inner conflicts.
- *Creating A Fertile Body*: to determine what the reproductive system needs.
- *Body Talk*: to identify any emotional factors which are affecting physical problems.

## Indirect approaches

Another way is to work indirectly or metaphorically with unconscious blocks to allow the resistance to be released without the client needing to gain conscious awareness. This more indirect approach can result in insight and tends to be less likely to result in re-traumatisation.

- *Fertility Garden*
- *Self-Integration Dissociation*
- *Fear Release*
- *IMR Signals*
- *Bird Cage Release*
- Metaphor/Storytelling.

## Homework

The following tasks enable the client to become aware of any inner conflicts or unresolved issues:

- Keep a journal and make a note of the negative thoughts that they have during the day. These thoughts are often very repetitive, and many people are unaware of them. This exercise produces conscious awareness of their thought patterns and may highlight any thinking that is ambivalent or conflicted about having children.
- *Cognitive Restructuring*: ask the client to notice times when they feel disturbed or upset about something relating to their fertility. Suggest that they make a note of what they were thinking which resulted in them feeling this way. Irrespective of whether they complete the next few steps

of the *Cognitive Restructuring* process, this information will provide you both with access to the unhealthy belief or past event relating to fertility that is unresolved.

## Age

Age is a significant factor in fertility as there does come a time in a woman's life when she will stop producing eggs and enter the menopause. While age does not affect men in quite the same way, an elderly man is more likely to have problems that affect his sperm quality and production. The problem, however, is that being 'too old' has become the so-called reason for fertility problems in many cases where the person is being viewed as a statistic rather than an individual.

The popularity and widespread publicity surrounding assisted reproductive technologies has made it seem as though every woman over the age of 35 is apt to have problems conceiving. But this just isn't true (Meldrum, 1993; Wood, 1992; Tan et al, 1992, pp. 1390–4). Simply being over 35 does not mean a woman is 'too old'. One woman who is 30 may have the reproductive age of a 45-year-old, while another woman who is 45 may have the reproductive age of a 30-year-old.

Some clients believe their age is a problem when there really are no grounds for this. When age becomes a limiting belief or a trigger for stress and causes a couple to feel that they must conceive urgently because time is running out, it is an issue that needs to be addressed and resolved.

Unfortunately I have heard many clients say they've been told by doctors, family or friends that 'time is running out' and they 'had better get a move on'. When I have asked them how they intend to 'hurry up' it often ends in laughter as they imagine ways to 'have sex quickly'. In other words, the belief that time is running out only adds to feelings of stress and anxiety since there is nothing they can do to 'hurry up'.

Another issue related to age that may need to be addressed is linked to self-blame. When people are told that their age may be a factor in their fertility problem they may blame themselves or their partner for not having tried for a baby sooner. After a client was told by her doctor that she had 'probably left it too late' she began to blame her husband for not being ready to have children sooner. During our session I asked her to become aware of the part of her that blamed her husband. She felt herself becoming progressively angrier as she accessed that part of herself. Her whole body became tense and hot and she was surprised at how strongly she was feeling this anger. I used EFT to tap on specific points on her body which allowed her to become fully aware of just how angry she felt.

As the feelings of anger rose in her body she started crying and told me that there were so many things that she wished she had said to him years ago but never did. As I continued tapping she moved from feeling angry at him to feeling angry at herself for not having told him how much she wanted to have a child. At the time she had felt that if she put too much pressure on him he might not agree to have children at all. Using EFT we were able to work back to an early experience, as a child with her father where he had denied her a toy which she desperately wanted because she had pestered her father too much for it. As she accessed this past experience and all the disappointment that she had felt as a little girl, I asked her adult self to step into the scene. Her grown-up self helped her see that although she had experienced this disappointment she was still free to say what it is she wanted, because if she didn't tell people what she wanted they might never know. Recalling this memory improved her understanding of her own behaviour and enabled her to let go of the blame and regret she had been feeling.

## Approaches

Age can present as an issue to be resolved in many different ways. The following techniques can be used to address some of the different issues connected to age:

- The *Doors Of Perception* is a good technique to increase awareness of how this belief is negatively affecting their mind and body.

- The *Primal Image* can be used to work with a particular body part that is perceived as being too old, such as the ovaries.

- *Parts Work* can be used to work through any regret, guilt or blame connected with leaving it too late.

- *Self-Integration Dissociation* enables clients to put up a protective barrier against negative messages about age, from doctors, friends and the media.

- *Cellular Memory Recall* to restore trust and confidence for those who have conceived in previous years.

- Time distortion gets clients to change their perception of time so that they can be more relaxed because they no longer feel time is running out.

- Direct suggestion to notice the vitality and youth in their body and to feel younger and better.

## *Previous termination*

Previous terminations of pregnancy are a source of great conflict for many women, especially when they discover some time later that they are having problems conceiving. The majority of women I have worked with did not have adequate support and help at the time of their termination and for many it remained a secret. Because of the secrecy that often surrounds terminations, it is important to reassure your client that what you discuss together is completely confidential.

While there are some women who have worked through their experience in the years following the termination, a large majority have just kept the lid on the box, so to speak. However, a previous termination isn't necessarily always an issue to address for fertility especially if the client has come to terms with it and they feel at peace with their choice. One woman told me that she mostly felt okay with it all, except during times of great disappointment, like when she got her period or heard a bad fertility test result. At these times she would notice that she tended to think that she was getting what she deserved and it was probably all happening because of what she had done. Although some aspects of her termination had been resolved it seems that she still had a deeply-seated belief that what she had done was wrong and she was being punished for it.

A person's belief system, whether that be cultural, spiritual or religious, may create an inner conflict about the decision they previously made to terminate a pregnancy. This inner conflict could result in unhealthy emotions such as guilt, shame, regret and anger at themselves or others. Clients who are conflicted about their choice may believe that their fertility problems are being caused or affected by their actions.

Some common beliefs a client may hold as a result include:

> *I don't deserve to have a baby.*
> *I've had my chance and Ive wasted it.*
> *I shouldn't have done it.*
> *I am being punished for what I did.*
> *I'm not ready to be a mother.*
> *It is my fault that we are not conceiving.*

Although I have been talking solely about women and terminations, this could also be an issue for men to resolve. A man came to see me for hypnotherapy because he and his wife had been diagnosed with unexplained infertility. He felt totally responsible for their diagnosis and told me that he had never told anyone that his girlfriend had fallen pregnant when he was 17. Although he was against abortions she decided to go ahead and have a termination. He felt helpless and ashamed by what they had done and had never told anyone about it before. We spent a lot of time talking about it and then used *Parts Work* and the *Healing White Light* to clear and release the shame and guilt he had been feeling.

Previous terminations are not always issues that clients consciously recognise as unresolved. It is not uncommon for women to 'sweep the termination under the carpet', or to 'forget about it'. When women have dissociated from their experience they may consciously believe and think that they feel okay about it all. While talking with a client about her termination she seemed very unaffected by it and told me that she knew she had done the right thing. During a trance session in which I had guided her into her *Fertility Garden*, her eyes suddenly shot open with fright and she told me that she had seen a young boy in her garden that looked just like her ex-boyfriend with whom she had accidently conceived. She told me that the boy looked about 10 years old, and then she burst into tears and said 'Which is the age he would be if I hadn't killed him.' These feelings of guilt had gone unacknowledged for the past ten years and had created a strong unconscious belief that she did not deserve to have a baby.

I feel that a vital part of this work is to allow women an opportunity to talk about their experience so that they can become conscious of how they really feel about it, as many men and women have not had the chance to speak about it openly and honestly.

## Questions

Below are some examples of questions which the therapist could ask:

- Were you well-supported and well-informed at the time?
- Did you take time off?
- Did you grieve at all? Did you feel you needed to?
- How did you feel about it? Do you still feel that way?
- Did any religious beliefs affect your choice or how you felt?

- Were you able to share your experience with anyone? Did they support you?

- If you had to do it again, would you?

- What did you learn?

- When you think about that termination now, how do you feel?

- Do you think this termination is having any effect on your fertility now?
(Domar and Kelly, 2002)

## Approaches

- *Parts Work*: working with the part responsible for the unhealthy belief or emotion resulting from the termination.

- *The Mirror Of Forgiveness*: to release any feelings of guilt and blame.

- *Self-Integration Dissociation*: to clear and let go of unhealthy beliefs and emotions about the termination that may be affecting fertility now.

- *Doors Of Perception*: to establish a healthy belief about their experience.

- *Healing White Light*: to cleanse and clear the mind and body from any disturbances or disruptions in the system resulting from the termination.

- *Rewind Technique*: if the termination was traumatic in any way or if they are having a strong emotional response when they think about it now.

- *Bird Cage Release*: to release the unhealthy emotions which are connected to the termination.

## Self-help tools

- Write a *letter of forgiveness* to yourself.
- Hold a *Ceremony To Say Goodbye*.
- *Affirmation:* to practise and reinforce the new belief and feeling.

## *Miscarriage*

Miscarriage is defined as the spontaneous loss of a pregnancy before 24 weeks' gestation when the foetus has a chance of survival outside the womb. Recurrent miscarriage is the loss of three or more pregnancies and occurs in about 1 in 100 women. It is important to recommend that women who have had three or more consecutive miscarriages see a gynaecologist for investigation and management of any treatable cause.

A miscarriage can often be a deeply traumatic and emotional experience, regardless of the stage of pregnancy it occurs. Miscarriage can be especially hard if the couple has been trying to conceive for a long time, or has suffered a miscarriage previously. The sense of loss following a miscarriage can be tremendous. Common reactions to the loss of a pregnancy are really no different to other forms of grief. Women who have miscarried may feel deep shock, numbness, guilt, a sense of helplessness, have difficulty sleeping and may find it difficult to concentrate on anything else.

## *Why does miscarriage happen?*

Miscarriage is the most common reason for gynaecological admissions into hospital in the UK. Most women do not discover the cause of their miscarriage, as miscarriages are rarely investigated unless a woman has had three or more.

It is thought that in most cases of early miscarriage the cause is a faulty chromosome – a one-off genetic problem in the baby that commonly does not happen again in future pregnancies. Less common causes of miscarriage include womb abnormalities, hormonal imbalance, infections such as listeria and rubella (German measles), auto-immune diseases such as Hughes Syndrome, and a weak cervix. Miscarriage is also more common in smokers, and as women get older. The miscarriage rate increases in women over the age of 30, but the fact remains that many women have successful pregnancies throughout their 30s, and into their early 40s (NHS, 2008).

## *Different types of miscarriage*

- Threatened miscarriage: bleeding in early pregnancy, where the cervix is found to be tightly closed. The pregnancy is most likely to continue.

- Inevitable miscarriage: bleeding in early pregnancy where the cervix is found to be open, suggesting that the pregnancy will be lost.

- Incomplete miscarriage: miscarriage has definitely started, but there is still some pregnancy tissue left in the womb. The cervix is usually found to be open.

- Complete miscarriage: pregnancy has been lost, the womb is empty and the cervix has closed.

- Missed miscarriage: pregnancy stopped a few weeks prior, but there was no bleeding at the time. This type of miscarriage usually causes a slight, dark-brown blood loss and the sudden end of normal pregnancy symptoms. It is sometimes called a blighted ovum.

## *Therapeutic approaches*

The most common cases I have worked with involving miscarriage include couples who have:

- Conceived easily but then gone on to miscarry. Since the miscarriage they have not been able to conceive again.

- Been trying to conceive for some time with difficulty, and then get pregnant but go on to miscarry.

- Experienced recurrent miscarriage.

- Have previously miscarried, and are now pregnant and filled with anxiety about having another miscarriage.

## *Working with clients who have experienced miscarriage*

There are many different aspects to working with clients who have experienced single or recurrent miscarriage and in this section I will address the following: future pregnancy, grief, beliefs, relationships and psychological/emotional causes. Sometimes miscarriage can be very traumatic, especially in cases where the mother's life has been threatened. In these cases the approaches and techniques suggested for trauma would be useful (Page 164).

*Future pregnancy*

If a couple experiences a miscarriage after they have been trying to conceive for a long time, it may be helpful to gently reframe their experience. You can do this by reminding them that the early pregnancy loss confirms that they can in fact conceive. In cases of miscarriage, reassure the woman that she still has a good chance of a subsequent successful pregnancy.

It may sometimes be necessary for clients to reduce their anxiety about future miscarriages as this may potentially affect their ability to conceive.

- *Cognitive Restructuring*: to challenge unhealthy beliefs relating to future pregnancy.

- Modify Thought Patterns: to interrupt anxiety-provoking thoughts.

- *Primal Image*: to create a womb that they know can carry a healthy pregnancy to full term.

- *Inner Guide*: to access their inner wisdom and resources.

- *Cellular Memory Recall*: to restore their confidence in their ability to conceive.

- Visualisation: enjoying a healthy thriving pregnancy and connecting with the positive emotions that they will experience during a healthy pregnancy.

- Direct suggestion: to develop greater trust in their body.

- *Self-Hypnosis*: for regular relaxation and positive visualisation.

- EFT: to clear any emotional disturbance which arises as they think about being pregnant.

Please refer to *Stage 6: Support* for information about how to work with clients who are pregnant and have previously experienced miscarriage (Page 164).

*Grief*

An important aspect of working with miscarriage is to enable the client to grieve and come to terms with their loss. Grief is a process that can't be rushed. In the same way that the autumn leaves take time to fall from the trees, coming to terms with the loss is a gradual letting go. Some clients need to be given permission to grieve because they feel that they can't because 'miscarriages happen all the time' or 'it wasn't even a baby yet' or 'there are far worse things that could happen,' and so on.

When a client tells me about their loss, I may ask them what they have done to commemorate it. Some people find it very helpful to have a ceremony. A couple who experienced a miscarriage at 15 weeks decided to put the scans, congratulation cards and other memorabilia into a small box and bury it in their garden. Another woman chose to plant a tree in her garden and another released a pink balloon into the sky. The client who had the balloon-releasing ceremony decided to repeat it on her baby's due date.

The expected due date is an important occasion to commemorate and could be seen as another opportunity for closure. Some people have told me that without even consciously realising that it was their baby's due date, they noticed that they felt very tearful or down and only later put two and two together. If a client's due date has not yet been reached I may draw their attention to it as an opportunity to say goodbye and mourn their loss.

It certainly seems that unresolved grief can affect a couple's ability to conceive. I can think of numerous cases that have resulted in pregnancy after a couple has allowed themselves to experience their feelings of loss. Using solution focused scales, the client can gauge the changes in their process and know when they have fully grieved. Using the *Primal Image* one client was able to see how full of grief her womb was. She saw this grief as a cold, damp, black weight inside her womb. She recognised that in order for her to have another baby, her womb needed to be empty and available, and at the moment it was occupied and filled with sadness. Each time she came to see me we revisited her womb to see what changes had occurred. When her womb was clear, light, warm and spacious she confirmed that she felt she had fully grieved and come to terms with her loss. Within two months she called me to tell me she had conceived. This is just one example of many women who have been through a grieving process and conceived within a few months.

Of course this is not always the case, and I certainly know of cases who have conceived without ever having shed a tear about their previous miscarriage. I do however think that addressing loss is an important part of creating mental, emotional and physical wellbeing.

The following techniques can be used when working with loss:

- *Self-Integration Dissociation*: the boundary can create a safe place in which to grieve. Once the boundary is strong and secure, the client breathes out any emotions they are holding onto, and breathes in the inner resources they need for coping with their grief.

- *Primal Image*: to work symbolically with the grief that they are holding in their womb.

- *Healing White Light*: to release and cleanse feelings of sadness and loss.

- *Safe Place*: to meet the baby and say goodbye.

- *Bird Cage Release*: to let go emotionally of the baby they have lost.

## Beliefs

It is important to address any unhealthy belief that the client holds as a result of the miscarriage. Some examples of what the client may be thinking include:

*I must have done something wrong, the miscarriage is my fault.*
*There is something wrong with me.*
*It's never going to happen; I'm never going to have a baby.*
*I have let everyone down, I'm such an idiot.*
*I don't trust my body.*
*I fail at everything I do.*

These kinds of thoughts perpetuate unhealthy feelings and can prevent clients from moving through the various stages of grief. Please refer to the information in *Stage 2: Balance* for working with beliefs (Page 59).

## Relationships

A miscarriage may be the first traumatic experience a couple has even gone through together. They could both be deeply affected but may deal with their emotions in different ways which can sometimes cause strain in the relationship.

With an early miscarriage, before the first scans, heartbeats and kicks, the pregnancy itself may well be more real to a pregnant woman than to her partner.

However, the fathers' feelings about miscarriage can often be overlooked, particularly if they are busy trying to 'stay strong' for their partner. As with most relationship difficulties, communication is the key to supporting each other and getting through it together.

*Psychological and emotional causes*

> *We have known for many years that emotional factors play a major part in the physiological sequences terminating in a spontaneous abortion. If organic factors have been ruled out, then careful attention must be given to the remaining psychological factors.*
>
> (Rossi and Cheek, 1994, p. 308)

Although it is possible that emotional factors are contributing to recurrent miscarriage, this situation needs to be handled very sensitively. For obvious reasons I would never suggest or imply that the client may somehow be to blame for their loss.

However, sometimes during trance the client may become aware of an emotional issue that is affecting their ability to hold on to the pregnancy. A client of mine who had experienced three previous miscarriages without any known cause became conscious of her own experience in utero. During a trance session, she spontaneously regressed to a time before her birth inside her mother's womb. During the session she became aware that her mother, who was unfortunately no longer alive and so was unable to verify this information, had been very sick during her pregnancy. My client felt that her mother's life had been under threat as a direct result of the pregnancy and that this experience was directly affecting her ability to maintain a pregnancy as she unconsciously believed that pregnancy meant risking death.

I worked with another woman who had come to see me because her relationship was falling apart. They had been through two miscarriages and were now struggling to conceive. As we worked together on restoring their relationship, she became aware that her lack of trust in her partner had been affecting her pregnancy. He had an affair in the early part of their relationship and she became aware of the part of her that was terrified of being left alone with a baby. She felt the pregnancies had naturally terminated because a part of her had felt too unsafe to bring a child into a broken relationship.

Aside from these kinds of spontaneous insights, I have not worked directly with the psychological and emotional causes of miscarriage as I feel it is of great importance that the client is not left feeling that the miscarriage is their fault.

## *Stillbirth and neonatal death*

The loss of a baby towards the end of pregnancy and any pregnancy loss after 24 weeks' gestation where the child was not born alive is referred to as a stillbirth. Neonatal death refers to the death of an infant within the first 28 days of life.

The death of a baby or infant is a devastating and tragic experience. Often the death is unexpected and the parents are unprepared for the experience. The effects of grief can be overwhelming and the couple may feel as if they will never cope.

The early moments of loss and how the baby's death is handled at the time can make a big difference to the clients' lasting memories of the experience. Most couples are given the opportunity to hold their baby, name him/her, have photographs taken and spend time saying goodbye. Often couples are referred for grief counselling. I have found that I tend to see people who have experienced this kind of loss after a significant amount of time has passed.

In cases of stillbirth or neonatal death my role has been:

- To support through any remaining aspects of grief

- To resolve any trauma related to their experience

- To prepare for future pregnancy.

Generally speaking, couples receive a lot of professional support after their loss, but the traumatic aspect of their experience is sometimes not addressed. For example, in one case the woman was suddenly told when she was in the middle of labour that there seemed to be a problem with the baby's heart beat. She was rushed into theatre where she was anaesthetised and the baby was born by Caesarean section. She came around from the anaesthetic to discover that her baby had died. In our conversations together she spoke about the smells, images and sounds that stayed with her from that day. The experience remained so vivid in her mind and filled her with such fear and anxiety that it continued to haunt her. Even though she had come a long way in terms of grieving her loss, the traumatic aspects of her experience still remained unresolved.

After working together for a number of sessions to build her inner resources and her capacity to relax deeply using hypnosis, we started to focus on resolving the trauma. When she told me that she felt ready to work through the trauma I asked her to spend some time at home writing her experience down, as if it were a movie that she was watching. She wrote about the experience from beginning to end with herself as a character in that movie. This let her step back from the intensity of the experience as she described it all. We then worked together using EMDR. Using eye movements and tapping we desensitised the peak moments, smells, sounds and images until she was able to recall them without the associated physiological response. After this work she noticed a significant difference in how she recalled the experience. She remarked how she was now able to notice her husband's presence and support throughout the whole experience and felt very grateful that she was not alone during this traumatic event.

In another example, I worked with a client who wanted to start trying for a baby after three years of grieving. Part of her goal for therapy was to be able to look forward to having a baby and be excited by the news that she was pregnant. She had done a lot of work to come to terms with her loss and felt that she had fully grieved for her son but was still unable to imagine herself with a baby.

Her son had died during labour and she had found it very comforting to be able to hold him after he had been born. She had two possible boys' names which she loved and decided to give him both names because at the time she really believed that she would never have another child. After we had been working together for some time, she realised that something significant had shifted for her because she had found another boy's name she really liked. Our work together focused on resolving the trauma of the birth and building a positive expectation through *Mental Rehearsal* and visualisation. We also used *Three Steps Forward* to reduce her anxiety about pregnancy.

More information about how to work with pregnant women who have experienced previous loss can be found in *Stage 5: Prepare* (Page 137) and *Stage 6: Support* (Page 157).

## *Menstrual health*

Menstrual health is an important part of female fertility and problems with the menstrual cycle may need to be resolved in order for conception to occur. According to some reports, 70% to 90% of women have recurrent menstrual problems. Many experience irregular periods and/or severely aggravated premenstrual symptoms. For some this can be so severe that it drastically affects their lives. For more information about the female reproductive system and the menstrual cycle please refer to Section D (Page 300).

Menstrual health problems include the following:

- Anovulation is a condition in which the ovary does not release a ripened egg each month and so with no egg available for the sperm to penetrate, a woman cannot become pregnant. Anovulation is a prime factor in infertility.

- Amenorrhoea is present when a woman fails to have menstrual periods. The condition is known as 'primary Amenorrhoea' when the woman has never menstruated; and 'secondary Amenorrhoea' if her periods cease after having been present for months or years.

- Dysmenorrhoea refers to painful menstruation and is classified as primary (from the onset of menstruation) or secondary (due to some physical cause and usually of later onset). Painful periods affect 40% to 70% of women of reproductive age. For about one in ten women the discomfort and pain is bad enough to interfere with their daily lives.

- Oligomenorrhoea refers to irregular or infrequent periods. Menstruation can occur anywhere from every six weeks to every six months. This is often associated with polycystic ovaries.

- Menorrhagia is recurrent heavy bleeding during menstruation.

- PMS (Premenstrual syndrome) is a cluster of symptoms, comprising physical and emotional changes, associated with the second part of the menstrual cycle. The essential feature of PMS is a cyclic pattern of severe emotional and behavioural symptoms. Symptoms begin one week before and cease within a few days after the onset of menstruation (American Psychiatric Association, 2000).

## Therapeutic approaches

Patients presenting with menstrual health problems and/or PMS require holistic treatment, which includes working with unresolved emotional issues. These are known to disrupt menstrual rhythm and normal hormonal balance, as we have seen with fertility problems. I have included some questions to ask the client, together with some more information about the different aspects of menstrual health, as well as some possible approaches.

## *Ideas for case history questions*

What are your emotional experiences during your menstrual cycle?
What symptoms do you experience prior to menstruation?
What are you confronted with Premenstrually?
When did you have your first period?
What was your family's attitude to your first period?
How did you feel about your first period?
What information were you given?
What messages about menstruation did you learn from your family?
Have you had a medical diagnosis?
What are your current levels of stress? (Rate them on a scale)
Do you use tampons, sanitary towels or something else?
What contraception have you used?
If you could create a sanctuary for yourself to go to during PMS what would it be like?
What do you want the days leading up to your period to be like?
What would you love to do Premenstrually and during menstruation if you didn't have to worry about others?
What do you like about being a woman? What don't you like?
How comfortable are you with your body?
How do you feel about talking about your menstrual cycle? Why?
What do you believe about your menstrual cycle?
How do you feel about this belief?
What do you tell yourself about your period?
What day of your cycle are you on today?
Is your cycle regular?
Have there been times when your cycle has been unusual?
What things would you like to do for yourself before/during your period?
What do you like about your cycle?
What don't you like about your cycle?
What's your favourite part of the cycle?
What's your least favourite part of the cycle?
Are the symptoms specific and regular like clockwork/or are they erratic and only happen sometimes?
If your PMS had a voice, what would it say to you?
What effect does your PMS have on your relationships?
If you had the courage to speak your truth, what would you say to: your partner/friend/community/family?

## A healthy attitude to menstruation

It is interesting to notice that menstruation is still one of the least publicly talked about subjects. Certainly in Western culture it is one of the few remaining taboos. When I ask women to tell me what they associate with periods, they tend to say things such as: embarrassing, painful, inconvenient, shameful, dirty, 'the curse', etc. Most of us have had very little positive information about menstruation and tend to see it as something that has to be tolerated. As a result a lot of women are in a continuing battle with their bodies and reject this part of their femininity.

This attitude tends to be compounded for women who have been trying to conceive for some time and have started to view their periods as a sign of failure and disappointment. After many months of unsuccessful conception, some women start to dread their next period. Each period signals another month of loss and the accumulated grief after many months of trying can sometimes feel overwhelming.

At the time of menstruation, the body is shedding and letting go of what it does not need so that it can prepare itself for the next cycle. It is a time of cleansing and renewal. Remind women that they can use menstruation as a time to really acknowledge their loss and feel their disappointment. Once they give themselves permission to do this, they can then prepare for the next cycle without the weight of unprocessed grief. Menstruation can also be seen as an opportunity to withdraw from the world and take time to be alone. Following the body's natural tendency to cleanse, let go and rest can be wonderfully therapeutic and also increase wellbeing at this particular time.

The client will develop a healthier attitude to the menstrual cycle if they value ovulation and menstruation equally. Sometimes clients need to be reminded that their period is a sign that their body is working, that it is a necessary and very beautiful part of their fertility.

Since our unhealthy attitude to menstruation is so deeply ingrained, I would suggest that clients read one or two of the books in the recommended reading list so that they may transform their thinking about their menstrual cycle (Page 300). Women who have altered their attitude to menstruation often report it as being a very empowering, significant and profound change in their lives and feel that on some level they are also healing a deep cultural wound.

*Approaches*

- *Healing White Light*: for women who have been trying to conceive for some time, menstruation may intensify feelings of sadness or grief at not having conceived, or of not being able to conceive. The *Healing White Light* clears and cleanses past cycles of grief and feelings of hopelessness.

- Reframe menstruation: for many women periods signify disappointment and/or failure. Gently remind your client that their period is a sign that everything is working, and that it signals the beginning of a new opportunity to conceive.

- *Primal Image*: As you think about your menstrual cycle now, what image comes to mind? How would that image change when your cycle is in a healthy, regular state?

- *Regression*: reframe their first menstrual period by going back to the start of menstruation and re-creating it as a healthy and supported experience. Address the needs that they had at the time which were not met. What would they have liked? Allow them to re-experience the onset of puberty as a powerful initiation into womanhood, in which they can feel honoured and respected.

- *The Storm Cloud*: to illustrate the cyclical nature of menstruation and encourage increased comfort with change.

## Listening and responding to biological rhythms

At different stages in the cycle we experience different feelings, perspectives and understandings. Because of the changing nature of our cycle we are constantly able to view the outer and inner world through different lenses. The physical, mental and emotional experiences of ovulation and menstruation are distinctly different. Cycling between these two worlds allow us to embody the polar opposites of life and death every month as we are reminded of the ever-changing cyclical nature of all things. A part of the wisdom of the menstrual cycle is that it's a reminder that there is a time for living and a time for dying, a time for creating and a time for letting go, a time for activity and a time for rest (Pope, 2001a).

When the natural changes brought about by the menstrual cycle are not acknowledged and followed, after a prolonged period of time, we are likely to experience negative psychological and physical effects and potential illness. Dr

Ernest Rossi, an expert in the field of chronobiology, studied an Ultradian cycle (a recurring cycle which is less than 24 hours long) and noticed how illness can result when our natural tendencies are not followed.

Dr Rossi studied an Ultradian cycle of 90 to 120 minutes during which there is a 20 minute drop in alertness and energy (Rossi, 2002). Many of the mind-body systems run on this same 90 to 120 minute Ultradian rhythm of peak activity followed by restoration. All the systems of regulation, including the nervous system, endocrine system and immune system, operate according to this 90 minute BRAC (Break Rest Activity Cycle). Even the brain follows this rhythm by shifting from left-brain dominance to right-brain dominance every 90 minutes.

Through Rossi's study of this BRAC he noted that ignoring the body's natural tendency for activity or rest leads to stress and possibly illness. According to him, this stress develops in four stages:

1. Lose concentration, feel tired, stretch, yawn, feel irritable.

2. Stress hormones such as adrenaline increase which give you a surge of energy during which time you can feel quite compulsive (compelled to do things).

3. Malfunction starts, you become accident prone, make spelling mistakes and bad decisions, have poor memory and become impatient.

4. Body starts rebelling, physical symptoms occur, possible illness results.

Rossi's work on the BRAC is significant since it explains how ignoring the body's natural tendencies during the menstrual cycle, which is an Infradian rhythm (a recurring cycle that is more than 24 hours long), may result in the above mentioned symptoms. Many, if not all, of the symptoms described above could just as easily be describing some of the typical Premenstrual symptoms (Pope, 2001).

A significant way to contribute to menstrual health is to increase our ability to listen and respond to what we need at different times of the cycle. There are, of course, many factors that influence menstrual health. By helping your client understand their cycle as more than just a biological process and something that needs to be listened and responded to, can create some profound changes.

*Approaches*

- Familiarise your client with the biological aspects of the menstrual cycle. The information provided in Section D (Page 300) will help your client get in touch with her body's natural tendencies at different times of the cycle.

- *Connect With Your Inner Body*: to help your client develop a deeper connection with her reproductive system. This is particularly useful for women who have lost faith in their body's ability to conceive.

- *Favourite Place*: this can be a useful resource for women to retreat into during menstruation, and can provide much-needed rest and relaxation.

- Visualisation: at menstruation imagine yourself deep within a cave where it is cosy, dark and quiet. You can continue to go about business as usual while a part of you remains snug and still inside your cave.

- Recommend rest during menstruation: listen to your body's natural tendency to slow down. In the days leading up to and during menstruation the following may be beneficial: *Meditation, Self-Hypnosis*, quiet walks, long baths, and *Creative Tasks*.

- *Self-Integration Dissociation*: to set clear and strong boundaries so that they can prioritise their needs and learn how to say no to others' demands.

- *Quick Body Scan*: to practise body awareness throughout the day, this is a good homework exercise to teach clients to become aware of their natural tendencies as they go through different stages of their cycle.

- *Nurturing*: as homework. This is especially important in the days leading up to and during menstruation.

## Working with PMS

Premenstrual syndrome (PMS) comprises of physical and emotional symptoms that are associated with the second part of the menstrual cycle. The variety of menstrual symptoms is enormous. It is important for each client to focus on what is being highlighted for them during this time. Look specifically at the emotional issues that arise, as these could serve as a guide to past unresolved issues. Since the menstrual cycle is a stress-sensitive system it can alert women to their own needs and serve as an early warning system for overall health. PMS could be understood as the body's way of delivering messages from the unconscious mind that we were are otherwise too busy to notice (Pope, 2001a).

The pre menstrum is like a magnifying glass, highlighting the things that we choose to ignore at other times in our cycle. Rather than viewing PMS as a problem to get rid of, it can be seen as signal from the unconscious mind that something needs to be addressed or tended to and that we may have needs that are not being met.

## Approaches

- Keep a journal: a daily record helps women become more aware of where they are in their cycle. Suggest that they keep track of which day of the cycle they are on, and ask them to pay particular attention each day to their physical symptoms, emotions, thoughts and behaviour.

- *Resource Gathering*: useful to do during pre menstrum as a way to gather resources for working with the feelings and things that come up at this time. Because women are much more sensitive and aware Premenstrually and during menstruation, some women may use food, drugs or other means to try to numb themselves and block out this awareness. Teach them how to tolerate their emotions, and be present to their experience. Give them access to resources, such as inner strength, so that they don't need to escape or resist their experience.

- *Creative Tasks*: if your client is finding it difficult to recognise what is going on for them Premenstrually, you could use art as a way for them to explore their experience more deeply. Give your client a relevant question to take home and create a drawing, collage or piece of art in response to it. Examples of questions could be:
    - What would I love to do Premenstrually and during menstruation if I didn't have to worry about others?
    - What am I confronted with Premenstrually? What is upsetting?
    - What am I confronted with as I bleed or am in pain?
    - What do I need emotionally?
    - What is my relationship with my body?
    - If I had the courage to express myself, what would I say to my boss/partner/mother-in-law?

- *Body Talk*: can be used to understand the purpose of the symptom and to develop greater body awareness.

## Ovulation and regular cycles

If a woman's cycles are irregular or she is failing to ovulate, the following techniques may be used:

- *Apposition Of Opposites*: to restore balance to the systems of the body.

- *Tune Into Your Body Clock*: to restore regularity and rhythm to the cycle.

- *Cellular Memory Recall*: to recall past times when the cycle has been healthy and regular.

- *Connect With The Inner Body*: to regulate the cycle.

- *Control Room*: find the control that governs the functioning of their hormonal system. Make the appropriate adjustments so that their hormonal cycle is working optimally.

- *Hypothalamus Meditation*: to reduce the effects of stress on the reproductive cycle.

For more information and inspiration about the menstrual cycle please refer to the recommended books in the reading list (Page 351).

## Parenthood

An often overlooked area in fertility is parenthood. Becoming a parent is a significant life change that involves great responsibility. Many people feel conflicted about wanting to become a parent. This ambivalence may negatively affect fertility.

> *One study showed that in women without any anatomical reason for infertility, the majority showed severe psychological conflict regarding the wish for parenthood.*
> (Benedek, 1953; Jeker et al, 1988)

Perhaps many women do not get pregnant because in their heart they do not want to. I believe that ambivalence is only a problem when it is not acknowledged or worked through.

How a client feels about parenthood can be affected by things such as childhood experiences, self-confidence and expectations and fears about how having children may negatively affect their life. It may be necessary to resolve past issues that are affecting how the client feels about becoming a parent.

## Questions

These two questions get the client to acknowledge some of the pros and cons of parenthood and may highlight any ambivalence or strong inner conflict about it.

- Why do you want a child?

- Why don't you want a child?

## Approaches

Please refer to *Preparation for parenthood* in *Stage 5: Prepare* (Page 149) as this will be useful in working with and addressing any ambivalence or concern about parenthood. The following techniques may be useful for resolving and working with specific issues about parenthood:

- *Parts Work*: to work with any inner conflict and to gather the resources needed.

- *Doors Of Perception*: to imagine a future with and without children. This will highlight any fears or give clarity about what the client wants.

- *Cognitive Restructuring*: to challenge any unhealthy beliefs about parenthood which may be causing internal conflict.

- *IMR Signals:* to locate a past event that is causing the ambivalence or conflict.

- *Fear Release*: to metaphorically address any fears about becoming a parent.

## *Stage 4: Enhance*

Stage 4 uses the conscious and unconscious mind to enhance fertility and the effectiveness of fertility treatments using guided imagery, visualisation and mental rehearsal. This may include working directly with fertility issues or working with any physical problems that may be affecting fertility, such as poor sperm morphology (a high percentage of abnormal sperm).

In this section, I explain how guided imagery, visualisation and mental rehearsal can affect physiology and create mental, emotional and physical change. I discuss how these approaches can be applied to physical problems affecting fertility and suggest a variety of techniques and ways of using them, along with some case histories.

**This section contains:**
- Visualisation approaches to enhance fertility
- Considerations when working with visualisation approaches
- Applications of visualisation approaches for fertility
- Visualisation scripts to enhance fertility
- Working with physical problems to enhance fertility.

## *Visualisation approaches to enhance fertility*

Guided imagery, visualisation and mental rehearsal are three terms which are largely interchangeable, although I use them to mean three slightly different things:

- Guided imagery (also sometimes referred to as guided visualisation) is a process in which the therapist leads the client through a specific visualisation, such as in the *Fertility Garden* or *Healing White Light*.

- Visualisation, on the other hand, is less directive and relies more on the client's ability to spontaneously generate their own imagery based on more general suggestions from the therapist, for example, the *Primal Image*.

- *Mental Rehearsal* is a visualisation process in which the client rehearses in their imagination the way they would like to think, feel and behave during a future event. Mental rehearsal refers to using our mind to 'replicate the experience of the actual doing of the thing' (Dispenza, 2007, p. 391).

Although all of the above-mentioned approaches contain the words 'visualisation' and 'imagery', which are both suggestive of seeing, they are actually intended to refer to the use of all modalities including hearing, smelling, tasting and touching/feeling. Different people will experience visualisation approaches in different ways, depending on their dominant modality. We know that some people are more likely to 'see' what is being evoked, while others may 'feel' or 'hear' it. Irrespective of how we use our inner senses, this process of actively engaging in a particular scenario instigates change.

The process of imagining by using our internal senses can create changes in the mind, body and behaviour. There is an intimate link between what we imagine and what becomes 'real'. There have many experiments and studies done to investigate the relationship between thoughts/imagination and physical/behavioural changes.

In one study a group of healthy five-year-old children were told a story about a magic microscope that showed how the immune cells in the body fight germs; they were also shown a film with glove puppets acting out the roles of different cells as policemen fighting off the germs. Saliva was collected before and after for analysis. After the experiment, the children's saliva was saturated with immunity substances at levels normal for fighting an infection (Shapiro, 2008, p. 80).

An article published in the *Journal of Neurophysiology* demonstrated the effects that mental rehearsal alone had on developing the neural networks in the brain (Pascual-Leone, 1995). The study included the comparison of two groups who were taught a sequence of notes on the piano, one group practised the sequence on the piano every day and the other group mentally rehearsed it. The group that only rehearsed the piano sequence mentally showed almost the same changes, involving the expansion and development of neural networks in the same specific area of the brain, as the participants who physically practised the sequence on the piano.

Mental rehearsal actually changes the physical composition of the brain in the same way that actually doing something would. Neural pathways form in the brain after repetitive thoughts, feelings and behaviours. When we have done something often enough it becomes, as it were, hard-wired into the brain. When neurons fire together they wire together. When patterns of thinking and behaving become hard-wired into the brain in this way, they become unconscious automatic responses. When we learn to drive a car, at first it is a very conscious process as we are creating new neural pathways, but after a period of practise, those pathways become hard-wired and we're able to drive without thinking about it (Dispenza, 2007, p. 48).

From these three examples alone we can see the far-reaching potential that visualisation and mental rehearsal can have for fertility. Below I have listed some of the ways in which these approaches can be applied to help enhance fertility and medical treatments.

## *Considerations when working with visualisation approaches*

- Visualisation is a natural function of the mind which we utilise on a day-to-day basis, often without realising it. When working with visualisation, explain what 'visualisation' means. Some people expect that visualisation requires them to be able to see things in their mind's eye as if they were watching a movie on their inner screen. However, only some people actually visualise in such graphic detail. Many others will experience it more as a general notion or a vague sense of something. Ask your client to recall the colour of their front door at home. Then point out that the way in which they accessed that information is what we mean by visualising. Another simple example of visualisation occurs when we go to the shop to buy a new piece of furniture. Before deciding to buy it we may spend a few moments imagining what it would look like in our home. If your client is clear on what is meant by visualisation, they are much more likely to engage in the process in a way that will bring them maximum benefit.

- An important component of guided imagery, visualisation and mental rehearsal is the state in which the client does this work. In order for guided imagery and visualisation to be effective it should always be accompanied by a state of mental and physical relaxation. A relaxed state of focused attention, which can be achieved through hypnosis, maximises the benefits and effectiveness of visualisation. When we access the trance state, our analytical left brain begins to 'switch off' and the right brain becomes more active as it generates inner imagery. Because the conscious critical functions are less active, this state allows us to bypass the limitations of the critical brain and to open up to new ways of perceiving and thinking. In the same way, the resistance which may be present in a normal waking state is less likely to be as active. Be aware that people who are in a high state of arousal (e.g. anxious) may find it more difficult to imagine things. For this reason I recommend that this work is preceded by some deep relaxation. For more information please refer to *Stage 2: Balance* (Page 55).

- Another important consideration when working with guided imagery is that you use suggestions and images that work for the client. Their interests and hobbies may provide some clues for this, as well as the descriptive and metaphoric language that they use. You could also simply ask your client if a particular concept or visualisation works for them.

- In order to maintain rapport when working with imagery or visualisation, ensure that you are matching your client: while they are in trance, ask them to describe *how* they are imagining something. Getting feedback during the trance session can help you to better facilitate the process and ultimately it is more likely to be effective.

- Finally, repetition is important. Encourage your client to use *Self-Hypnosis* for visualisation on a daily basis. For those who are able to visualise quite easily, I recommend that they take a few moments throughout the day to revisit those mental images. Positive visualisation can help to give people a healthy mental focus and offers them a good alternative to worrying. A man who spent a lot of time worrying about his fertility problems gave me the idea of suggesting that each time he noticed himself worrying he could recall that positive mental image that he had accessed during the session. His persistent worry served as a great cue for him to do some positive visualisation. A similar suggestion can support women who are going through the IVF two week wait. Irrespective of how you go about it, the important thing is that the client revisits the visualisation/mental rehearsal on a regular basis.

## *The applications of visualisation approaches for fertility*

Visualisations can be used as a means to communicate with the body and create mental, emotional and physiological changes. Visualisation can be used to:

- Heal specific physical conditions such as fibroids, endometriosis and poor sperm morphology.

- Understand the body and gain insight into symptoms and conditions as well as to find out what the body may need for healing.

- Increase the healing process which can be useful for things such as surgical recovery and so on.

- Increase body awareness. For example, the *Body Talk* script can be used to develop awareness and to understand what the body is trying to communicate through its symptoms.

- Imagine egg fertilisation, implantation and the successful outcome of treatment which can help keep a positive mental focus and reduce worry.

- Imagine the womb as a safe, supportive place and see the embryo growing into a healthy, strong baby. This is especially helpful for women who have had previous miscarriages.

Imagery, metaphor and symbols are the language of the unconscious mind. Guided imagery can be used as a way to:

- Communicate and influence the part of the mind that regulates bodily functions and unconscious body processes (including conception).

- Enhance medical treatments in many different ways. Use guided imagery throughout medical treatments and specifically during embryo transfer because it helps to relax the uterine muscles and increase blood flow to this area. This has been shown to increase the chances of successful implantation (Levitas, 2006).

*Mental Rehearsal* can be used to rehearse new behaviours and future successes. *Mental Rehearsal* can:

- Help improve enjoyment and spontaneity of sex. This is especially important when sex has become all about trying to get pregnant.

- Build confidence and trust in your body by imagining being pregnant or holding your baby.

- Prepare for future situations and practise ways of responding and coping. This is especially useful during IVF.

- Prepare the client mentally and emotionally for the changes that parenthood will bring.

- Build positive expectations for women who have previously miscarried, for their next pregnancy. This also reduces worry and anxiety.

With just about all of my clients I tend to use some form of visualisation to enhance fertility. In some cases, visualisation approaches can be the main focus of the treatment while in others it may be just one of many essential ingredients. For example, the client's goal and circumstances may mean that the main focus of therapy is on resolving a particular issue and *Stage 4: Enhance* may be used more as 'the icing on the cake', so to speak.

When I work with clients who are only able to see me for a few sessions I use guided imagery and visualisation as a simple and direct way of helping them enhance their fertility. The combination of goal setting (*Stage 1: Outcome*), relaxation (*Stage 2: Balance*) and visualisation (*Stage 4: Enhance*) can also be very effective.

## *Case study: making the most of limited time*

A woman from abroad came to see me while she was in London for a few days on business. We were able to schedule two sessions together in the time she had available. In the first session, we clarified her goal for therapy which was to believe that her body was capable of carrying a baby. Silvia had been diagnosed with endometriosis a few years before and had since been for surgery to have it removed. Her doctor had confirmed that the endometriosis was no longer a problem and that she should now be able to conceive. Despite this she still imagined that her womb was overcrowded with the endometriosis and that she would not be able to fall pregnant. As part of her goal I asked her to tell me how she would be imagining her womb when she did believe that her body could carry a baby. She said that she would imagine her womb as open and available and feel that there was enough space inside it for a baby to grow. This, along with some other details that she gave me, became the seeds for the visualisation work that we did together.

In the first session we focused on creating a clear goal state (*Stage 1: Outcome*) and doing some deep relaxation (*Stage 2: Balance*). I also taught Silvia how to access this state of relaxation on her own. In the second session (*Stage 4: Enhance*) I used the *Primal Image* so that she became more aware of how she perceived her womb. She described it as an overgrown garden which had run wild and become overcrowded and unmanageable. Weeds had overrun the garden and there was no space for beautiful flowers and plants to grow. The garden appeared dark, cramped and uninviting. I asked her, in trance, if you knew that you were able to carry a baby, how that garden would be different. She said that the garden would be clear of weeds, and the ground would be turned and softened and ready. It would be spacious, sunny and inviting so that you felt as if you wanted to spend time relaxing there. I then asked Silvia to imagine that she was an accomplished gardener with all the right tools and equipment needed for the job, and to go into the garden and begin clearing some of the weeds and undergrowth. I suggested that she may even find it very satisfying and relaxing to clear and de-weed her garden.

When she felt satisfied that it was done, I suggested that she till and soften the soil so that it would be ready for any new seeds which might be planted. Since gardens are living, dynamic things, I suggested that she return to this garden every day to tend it, to prune anything that needed to be cut back or simply to rest and relax in the warm and inviting place that she had created. I completed the trance session with some future orientation / *Mental Rehearsal* so that she could see herself thinking, feeling and behaving in a way that told her she did believe it was possible for her to carry a baby.

After the session I recommended that she practise her self-hypnosis relaxation every day, and take the time to revisit her 'womb garden' to do the necessary work or simply to relax there. Silvia went on to conceive a few months later and she is a good example of how effective visualisation and guided imagery work can be.

## *Visualisation scripts to enhance fertility*

Section C (Page 181) contains a collection of visualisation scripts for use in enhancing fertility and increasing the likelihood of natural conception and successful assisted fertility treatment. These include:

- *Primal Image*
- *Inner Guide*
- *Creating A Fertile Body*
- *Healing White Light*
- *Healing Green Light*
- *Fertility Garden*
- *Control Room*
- *Safe Place / Favourite Place*
- *Pseudo-orientation / Future Pacing / Mental Rehearsal*
- *Conception*
- *The Big Race*
- *Connect With The Inner Body*
- *Embryo Transfer*
- *Implantation*

- *IVF preparation*
- *Self-Hypnosis*: to visualise or mentally rehearse on a daily basis.

## Working with physical problems to enhance fertility

Physical symptoms are often a signal from the body that something needs to be attended to. Trance states of deep inner absorption assist clients in understanding the messages from their body. Use guided imagery and visualisation to help the client understand and possibly improve any physical symptoms that might be affecting fertility. The following case studies illustrate how visualisation approaches can improve symptoms and enhance fertility.

### Case study: visualisation for high FSH

A vibrant young artist came to see me after tests showed that her FSH levels were abnormally high. Melissa and her husband wanted to have IVF, but had been told that her FSH levels indicated that she was unlikely to respond well to the treatment. Unless Melissa's hormone levels came down they'd be unable to have assisted fertility treatment.

Understandably, she felt devastated by the news and started to believe that she may never be able to have children. She came to see me because she had been feeling really low and increasingly anxious.

After we had completed the necessary and essential work of goal setting (*Stage 1: Outcome*) and restoring mental and emotional balance (*Stage 2: Balance*) we began to focus on *Stage 4: Enhance*. During a trance session I guided her on a journey to meet her *Inner Guide,* with whom she could talk and seek advice and guidance about her physical condition. Being an artist, she had a magnificent visual capacity and described her inner guide to me in graphic detail. When she asked her guide to help her restore her fertility, he showed her a photograph of herself as a young girl holding up an award that she had received at school. When I asked Melissa what that photograph meant to her, she began to cry and told me that she had always tried to do well to please her mother, but no matter what she did it never seemed to be good enough. Her inner guide got her to understand that her desire to 'achieve' and 'succeed' and 'be perfect' was contributing to her high FSH levels.

In the following session I combined *Stage 2: Balance* (resource building) and *Stage 4: Enhance* using the *Healing White Light* visualisation to bring in the resources needed to 'accept herself more' and feel 'good enough', and to clear the 'old patterns of behaviour' that were creating unnecessary stress in her system. I asked Melissa to imagine her body's natural balance returning as the light brought acceptance and transformation.

Along with the *Healing White Light* visualisation to enhance fertility, we did further work on addressing her core belief (*Stage 3: Resolve*) that she was 'not good enough'. Over a number of sessions, using a combination of EFT, *IMR Signals* and *Mental Rehearsal* she began to notice some significant changes in her thinking. Her regular FSH level tests became more variable and over time began to stabilise within a more healthy range.

## Case study: fibroids

Uterine fibroids are tough, fibrous, non-cancerous lumps that grow in the uterus and can sometimes affect fertility. In Kathryn's case, she had been offered surgery to remove the fibroids but had decided that she would prefer to try to heal it in a less invasive way first.

Once we had clarity on her goal, (*Stage 1: Outcome*) I did some deep relaxation and taught her how to enter a trance state on her own (*Stage 2: Balance*). Having done a lot of yoga and meditation she found it very easy to enter trance and so I suggested that she could practise entering this state and becoming more sensitive to her body.

In the following session, while in a light trance, I asked her to tune in to her body and become aware of the fibroids. Along the lines of the *Primal Image*, I asked her to identify the shape, size, colour, texture, and temperature of the fibroids. Following the concepts in the *Body Talk* script I asked Kathryn to listen, see and sense what the fibroids were trying to tell her. She chose not to verbalise her insights but gave me a head nod when she was done.

After the session (*Stage 4: Enhance*) she told me that the fibroids appeared to her as a huge overcrowded tower block, like the ones you might see in an underprivileged part of town. She could hear people arguing and shouting inside the building, and was aware of litter lying around accompanied by an unpleasant smell. She felt that the fibroids were trying to tell her that her system was overloaded and toxic and in need of some cleansing.

In the next session we continued to work with *Stage 4: Enhance* and while in trance I asked her to revisit her fibroids. Using visualisation, I suggested that she find a creative way of 'cleaning up' the tower block. Kathryn imagined using a giant vacuum cleaner that sucked up all the litter and rubbish. She then used a silver hose to clear out all the angry inhabitants along with all their clutter. She imagined it all being washed away leaving the building clean, spacious and fresh.

I then asked her if there was anything else she felt she needed to do to restore her fertility. She realised that, having cleared the tower block of all the inhabitants, there was in fact no need for the building to remain, so she found a blue hose which blew a powerful stream of air towards the building causing it to disintegrate.

I suggested that she continued to use *Self-Hypnosis* every day to revisit the land where the building had been and make any adjustments or changes that may be needed. When Kathryn came back for her next session she told me that each time she returned there, she had planted some seeds so that the land could be rejuvenated and revived.

Some months later I discovered that fibroids are caused by excess oestrogen levels, which can, in part, result from an excess of synthetic hormones in the system, coming from the use of hormone therapies such as the contraceptive pill. It was interesting to me that, without consciously knowing this, Kathryn had intuitively detected that excess toxicity was causing/maintaining the fibroid. Upon learning this she decided to support her mind-body work by following a good detoxification diet.

The final piece of work we did together focused on restoring balance to her endocrine system (*Stage 2: Balance*) using the *Apposition Of Opposites* technique. Although it took almost nine months, using a combination of hypnosis and diet, her fibroids shrank and no longer affected her fertility.

## Stage 5: Prepare

Preparing for any future event requires that you have adequate information about the event so that you know what to expect, and that you are equipped with all the tools and resources that you may need to handle that event in a way that you feel comfortable with.

*Stage 5: Prepare* is the preparation stage of the *Fertile Body Method* and can include educating the client about an upcoming event, (such as pregnancy, birth, parenthood, IVF) and encouraging them to find out more about it through reading, internet surfing, and talking to others. The education that the therapist provides should be factual and should also provide a positive expectation and healthy reframe about the upcoming event. Preparation can also include the use of hypnotherapeutic tools, self-help tools and/or tasks carried out between sessions. As can be seen in the case study examples, it is the work done in Stages 1 to 4, combined with *Stage 5: Prepare* which ultimately helps the client feel more prepared.

**This section contains:**
- Preparation for pregnancy
- Preparation for birth
- Preparation for parenthood
- Preparation for medical treatments.

## *Preparation for pregnancy*

Preparation for a healthy, happy pregnancy is especially important for those who have previously had problems during pregnancy or who are particularly anxious about miscarrying. For those who are worried about miscarriage and loss, it may be hard for them to acknowledge the pregnancy until such time as they feel it is 'safe' to do so. Often the 12-week scan is a milestone that many women look forward to. For those who have lost babies at later dates they will tend to look beyond that time as a 'safe zone'. Due to their past experiences, some women fear that they could lose their baby at any time during or after the pregnancy. Concern about recurrent loss is very normal and natural. Sometimes, however, concern escalates into anxiety, fear and panic.

If you have been able to work with your client prior to conception, you may have been able to resolve (*Stage 3: Resolve*) some of their past miscarriages. This should help reduce their level of anxiety during pregnancy. The work done in *Stage 2: Balance* enables your client to access the inner resources they may need to cope with any possible problems that may occur during the current or future pregnancy. If your client believes that they can cope with another loss they are less likely to become extremely anxious during a subsequent pregnancy. For this reason, building their strength and resourcefulness is vital.

In cases where women have miscarried one or more times and begun to fear becoming pregnant, just the idea of a positive pregnancy test may be enough to create panic. A client once told me that her biggest fear would be to find out that she was pregnant, because then she knew she would be faced with the possibility of another miscarriage. She recognised that this put her in a difficult position as her greatest desire at that time was to have a baby. Part of her goal for therapy was to be able to get excited about the possibility of being pregnant, she wanted to be able to think about pregnancy as being exciting. The work we did together to bring some closure to her past miscarriages, combined with pseudo-orientation and resource building, helped her to look forward to getting pregnant again.

For information about how to support and work with clients who are already pregnant when they come to see you, please refer to *Support during pregnancy* in *Stage 6: Support* (Page 163).

Generally, preparation for pregnancy is about building a positive expectation as well as giving the client tools to manage any anxiety or fear that may arise when they think about being pregnant. Please refer to *Anxiety* in *Stage 2: Balance* for more information on how to manage anxiety (Page 73).

*Case questions / education*

- Encourage your client to find out about the different stages of pregnancy and what they're likely to experience.

- Find out what their expectations of pregnancy are.

- Address any fears or concerns that they may have about pregnancy. This is particularly important if the client has experienced previous miscarriage. The case study below gives an example of this.

- Ask them what would help them become more relaxed during this pregnancy.

- Find out what kind of pregnancy they would like to have, and what they are most looking forward to.

- Scale any disturbance/goal state. For more information please refer to *Working with scales* (Page 35).

*Approaches*

- Direct suggestion: can be used to direct their attention towards some of the positive signs of pregnancy. Some clients become obsessed with every twinge or ache and fear that it is a bad sign. Direct suggestion gets them to focus on the natural changes that are happening in their body and the positive signs that their pregnancy is progressing well.

- *Resource Gathering*: mobilising inner resources so that they feel they can cope no matter what occurs during the pregnancy.

- *Three Steps Forward*: to reduce the anxiety associated with pregnancy. This visualisation technique can be taught and done in *Self-Hypnosis* daily before and during pregnancy.

- *Fear Release*: to let go of specific fears and concerns that they have associated with pregnancy.

- *Pseudo-orientation / Future Pacing*: to the 12-week scan, to hear the foetal heart beat. This builds a positive expectation. Pseudo-orientation to other points in the pregnancy should be done sensitively as some women may find it too difficult to imagine themselves beyond a certain point in the pregnancy.

- *Primal Image*: to see a womb that is safe and secure and able to support a pregnancy until birth.

- *Inner Guide*: to receive advice and reassurance from their guide for a healthy pregnancy.

- Visualisation for pregnancy: mentally rehearsing a positive pregnancy.

- *Cellular Memory Recall*: to recall positive past pregnancies.

- EFT: to reduce specific fears associated with pregnancy and can be taught as a self-help tool to reduce anxiety.

- EMDR: to desensitise any images, beliefs or physical sensations that come up when they think about being pregnant.

*Self-help tools*

- *Self-Talk SUDS*: to reduce negative self-talk which is producing anxiety about the pregnancy.

- *Affirmations*: to maintain a positive mental focus.

- *Mini-Break Anchor*: to manage anxiety or fear.

- EFT: to reduce anxiety about pregnancy.

- *Self-Hypnosis*: to practise the *Three Steps Forward* technique. This is best done on a daily basis as long as the client is experiencing any anxiety about the pregnancy.

## Case study: preparing for pregnancy

A couple who had experienced two previous miscarriages contacted me for hypnotherapy treatment when they began trying for the third time. I saw them both individually to address their understandable concern about a recurrent miscarriage. In my session with Victoria she explained that she was dreading being pregnant again because she felt she couldn't handle another miscarriage. Her previous pregnancy had been wrought with anxiety and every time she felt any kind of sensation in her body she feared that it might be signalling a problem. She felt that being in such an anxious state may be contributing to her inability to carry to full term. Victoria had been stuck in a vicious circle of 'feeling anxious about feeling anxious' which she didn't know how to get out of. She wanted to be able to enjoy her pregnancy and feel more relaxed during it.

Many people fall into the spiral of worrying about being anxious during their pregnancy. Reassure women that it is normal, given their previous experience, to be concerned about losing their baby during pregnancy. Resisting or fighting any feelings that arise tends to propagate and heighten stress and tension. For this reason I suggested that she give herself permission to be a little anxious and concerned from time to time and know that it's okay and normal. Through allowing and integrating her feelings instead of resisting them, they were much more likely to pass.

In *Stage 1: Outcome* I asked Victoria a number of solution focused questions to get a full picture of what an enjoyable, relaxed pregnancy would be like for her. I also asked her to identify what would help her enjoy her pregnancy more.

Victoria was a very creative art teacher and had access to a wealth of art material. Once we had created a SMART, healthy goal for therapy, I suggested that she create a piece of art that captured her goal state and some of the resources that she had identified. At the time, the idea of an enjoyable pregnancy seemed to be a far-fetched possibility for her. I gave her the *Creative Task* as a way to encourage her to spend more time engaging in the possibility of an enjoyable pregnancy.

She created a magnificent sculpture of a heavily pregnant woman with one hand resting lovingly on her belly. In her other hand she was holding an apple. The expression on the sculpture's face was one of total bliss. Behind the sculpture lay a small pile of autumn leaves.

She described the leaves as being symbolic of her putting all her past losses behind her, as she looked forward to having her baby. The apple, she said symbolised the strength she would need to stay in the present moment during the pregnancy rather than fall back into the fear of losing another baby. I asked her to keep this sculpture in a place where she would see it every day.

During *Stage 2: Balance* I focused on teaching her deep relaxation using self-hypnosis so that she knew how to access a calm, relaxed state on her own. I taught her the *Self-Talk SUDS* so that she could become more aware of her inner dialogue and make changes to the way that she was thinking to increase relaxation on a daily basis. These two tools would be very helpful for her during pregnancy as a way of managing her mental, emotional and physical state. At the same time, they increased her current level of relaxation so that we could work more effectively together.

The next part of *Stage 2: Balance* was aimed at developing and building the inner resources that she might need to feel that she could cope with the possibility of another miscarriage. I asked her to rate her current level of anxiety about having a miscarriage, which she scored at -10 out of -10 on the scale.

Using the *Resource Gathering* technique she was able to access a positive past experience in which she had the strength to deal with and overcome a very difficult situation in her life. Before finishing the session I asked her to visualise her sculpture and notice how bright, colourful and juicy the apple now appeared. After the session I asked her to scale her anxiety levels and she felt that they had come down to a -5 on the scale.

In *Stage 3: Resolve* we worked with EFT to resolve some of the anxiety that she was feeling about the possibility of having another miscarriage. She knew that having some concern about having another miscarriage would be fine, but at the moment her fear felt so overwhelming that it was affecting her whole life. She said that when she was a -1 (on the -10 to 0 scale) that would indicate a 'normal' level of concern which would allow her to enjoy a pregnancy as best she could given the circumstances. Using EFT, her anxiety levels came down to a -3 in the first session, and were down to a -1 by the end of the second session of EFT.

With her levels of anxiety significantly reduced, and her inner resources more accessible, we were able to begin to prepare her for an enjoyable

> pregnancy (*Stage 5: Prepare*). The *Primal Image* helped her develop more confidence in her body. She metaphorically moulded soft clay earth around her womb and infused it with a warm comforting colour. Each night before going to sleep she would spend ten minutes in a trance state, revisiting her warm, safe womb. She also continued to practise her deep relaxation on a regular basis and found that overall she felt much calmer and more relaxed.
>
> And finally, to prepare her mentally and emotionally for an enjoyable pregnancy I asked her to visualise her future pregnancy and I included suggestions based on what she had identified for her goal state.
>
> By the end of our six sessions together, she felt prepared for pregnancy and equipped to manage her emotional state. Although she was not yet pregnant she felt she had achieved her goal for therapy because she was actually looking forward to getting pregnant. Importantly, she also believed that she and her husband were in a much better place to be able to deal with things should anything go wrong.

## *Preparation for birth*

Birth preparation is a very important part of fertility work. The *Fertile Body Method* is designed to help people from pre-conception, through pregnancy until after the baby is born. However, the information provided in this section only offers a few key pointers and suggestions for birth as I feel that birth preparation really requires a book unto itself.

Childbirth education is a crucial part of birth preparation and will be available to your client in books, websites, from friends and through childbirth educators. The delivery of this information, as well as the words used to describe particular aspects of birth, will play a major role in the woman's perception of birth. Good childbirth education provides factual information and instils confidence in the woman's natural ability to comfortably birth a baby. This is important as a woman giving birth naturally really needs to understand and trust her body.

Please refer to the Resources section for more information about childbirth education, hypnosis for childbirth training and recommended books (Page 351). In some cases it may be best to refer your client to someone who specialises in hypnosis for childbirth if this is not an area in which you work.

Preparation for birth is likely to be of particular importance if the client has had a disturbing previous birth experience. With previous birth trauma or a fear of giving birth, the work done in *Stage 3: Resolve* can be combined with *Stage 5:*

# The Fertile Body Method

*Prepare* to increase the client's confidence and comfort for birthing her baby. This section contains some educational information for the client, as well as some possible approaches and self-help tools.

## Education

To prepare women for giving birth, explain how thoughts and emotions can negatively impact on the body during birth. Below is an explanation:

> *There are three layers of muscles in the uterus. The outer layer consists of vertical muscles that go up the back and over the top of the uterus where they are at their strongest. The inner layer consists of muscles that are horizontal and circle around the baby. These circular muscles are thickest just above the opening, of the uterus, which is called the cervix.*
>
> *In order for the cervix to open and permit the baby to easily move down through and out of the uterus into the vagina, these lower, thicker circular muscles have to relax and thin. During birth the vertical muscles tighten and draw up the circular muscles at the neck of the uterus, causing the edges of the cervix to progressively thin and open. Then, in a wave like motion, the vertical muscles shorten and flex to nudge the baby down, through and ultimately out of the uterus.*
>
> *When the birthing mother is in a state of relaxation the two sets of muscles work in harmony and the mother will experience very little discomfort. The surge of the vertical muscles draws up, flexes and expels; the circular muscles relax and draw back to allow this to happen. The cervix thins and opens. Birthing occurs smoothly and easily.*
>
> *Fear has a physiological effect on the normal process of labour and its harmful effects can delay, stall and restrict labour. When a mother approaches labour feeling fearful, her body moves into a defensive state (the fight-or-flight response), releasing stress hormones and activating the sympathetic nervous system. Blood is directed away from the uterus towards parts of the body that may be used in defence, such as the arms and legs. This limited supply of oxygen rich blood to the uterus causes the lower circular fibres of the uterus to tighten and constrict. The outer vertical muscles continue to draw up in waves during contractions but are met with the resistant and constricted lower circular muscles causing pain and discomfort. This fear response results in the cervix remaining thick and closed. This tension not only causes pain to the mother, the baby's oxygen supply becomes restricted and the pressure of the tight muscles may cause discomfort to the baby. Dr Grantly Dick-Read, a British obstetrician who is regarded by many as*

*the father of the natural childbirth movement, refers to this as the Fear–Tension–Pain syndrome (Dick-Read, 2005).*

*If the mother is profoundly relaxed, then labour discomfort is not a necessary component of childbirth. Relaxation helps avoid the Fear–Tension–Pain (FTP) syndrome.*

## Hypnotic tools

- Direct suggestion: to trust in her body's ability to birth her baby, to follow her body's natural instincts and to work with her baby during the birthing process.

- *Pseudo-orientation / Mental Rehearsal*: mentally rehearsing the birth of the baby while feeling calm, relaxed and in control.

- *Fear Release*: to let go of specific fears and concerns that she may have associated with giving birth.

- *Safe Place / Favourite Place*: to create a safe place that the woman can access during labour.

- *Teach Self-Hypnosis*: this is one of the key skills a woman needs to develop so that she can easily access this state of deep inner absorption. This will allow her to feel more relaxed during the birthing process and to connect more easily with her birthing body.

- *Resource Gathering*: for a particular quality that the woman would like to have access to during her birth, for example 'trust' or strength.

- Visualisation for pregnancy: mentally rehearsing a positive pregnancy.

- EFT: to reduce specific fears associated with birth and be taught as a self-help tool to reduce anxiety.

*Self-help tools*

- *7:11 Breathing*: through regular practise of breathing exercises such as the 7:11 the client can learn to greatly reduce stress through stimulating the relaxation response of the parasympathetic nervous system and minimises the habitual sympathetic stress response.

- EFT: to reduce anxiety or fear about birth.

- *Mini-Break Anchor*: can be used to reduce anxiety at any point during the pregnancy, for example when the pregnant woman feels a twinge or cramp.

- *Self-Hypnosis*: for focus, relaxation and connection to her birthing body.

- *Affirmations*: repetitive affirmations for a positive pregnancy and gentle birth encourages a chain of beliefs, feelings and experiences that can be encouraging and supportive during birth.

# The Stages of Treatment

## *Case study: preparing for birth*

Fears about giving birth can stem from all kinds of past experiences. Sonja, at the age of 33, still consciously remembers an event that deeply disturbed her at the age of 4.

She remembers seeing a woman on TV screaming and crying as she gave birth. She could still recall the horror that she felt at what this woman was going through and the bloody images remained imprinted in her mind.

Sonja came to see me after she had been diagnosed with unexplained infertility, thinking that this memory may be the cause of her problems. As I later found out, she had in fact conceived about a week before coming to see me but was not aware of this at the time of our first appointment. After the first session she returned to tell me that she was already pregnant (and joked about how powerful hypnotherapy must be!). Now more than ever she felt she needed to address her fear of giving birth. Her goal for therapy was to feel comfortable about giving birth so that when she thought about it she no longer recalled the TV scene, but instead imagined herself in a calm, tranquil environment giving birth to her baby. In *Stage 1: Outcome* of the treatment we scaled her goal and gathered some more specific information about how she would know when she had reached her goal for therapy.

In *Stage 2: Balance* we did some deep relaxation using the *Safe Place* visualisation technique. I taught her this visualisation as a *Self-Hypnosis* exercise and she agreed to practise it every day. The *Safe Place* had the dual purpose of relaxation and building safety. Given that the initiating event happened while she was watching TV, I thought that the *Rewind Technique* would be an apt and effective way of resolving the emotional disturbance she had about childbirth. The *Safe Place* would provide a resource state that she could access, should she need to, during the *Stage 3: Resolve* work to follow.

In the following session I asked Sonja to describe to me every detail that she could recall about the day of the TV programme, and the programme itself. As she described it to me, I asked her, at various intervals, to rate her level of disturbance from -10 to 0 (with 0 being no disturbance). Once she was done, I asked her to identify the moment of peak intensity from that memory. She said it was the moment when she realised that the screaming and blood was because the woman was giving birth to a baby, she visually recalled it as the moment when she saw the bloody baby. She rated this peak moment as being a -10 out of -10 on the disturbance scale. I asked her to describe the sensations she was feeling in her body now as she thought about that peak moment. She felt it in her tummy as a, 'knotted sick nausea'. Getting people to gauge their disturbance on a scale and in their body provides useful information; firstly it tells you if they are actually tuning in to the disturbance and secondly it gives you two measures for change. I then suggested that she put that memory 'out the door', and that she didn't need to think about it any more.

Using the *Safe Place* to once again induce relaxation and create feelings of safety, we began the process to resolve this memory. After the desensitisation of the *Rewind Technique*, and still in trance, I asked her to bring that peak scene onto the screen in front of her. She rated her response as being about a −2 and said that her stomach felt 'okay'. After the session I suggested that she spend some time looking on the internet for video clips of positive, comfortable birth experiences. She liked the idea, and I felt that she needed to find some alternative images for birth. This homework task began *Stage 5: Prepare*.

Sonja returned two weeks later, grinning from ear to ear. She couldn't believe what she had found on the internet and felt very excited about the possibility of birth being an intimate and sensual experience. She had also bought a couple of books which I recommended (please refer to *Recommended reading* for books on pregnancy and childbirth, Page 351) and was beginning to see how it was in fact possible to enjoy giving birth. Combining the *Safe Place* induction (for reinforcement) and *Pseudo-orientation* she began to imagine herself having a positive birth experience, just as she had seen other women having in the video clips she watched. I suggested that she could take a few moments each day to gently rub her belly in a loving way and each time she rubbed her belly her confidence and trust in her body would grow. This cue would help her to maintain the changes, *Stage 6: Support*. Along with her regular *Mental Rehearsal*, I recommended the daily exercise of rubbing her belly as a way to maintain and build her trust in her body.

She had reached her goal for therapy and felt inspired to find out as much as she could about natural childbirth. Our work together became a platform for her to go on and equip herself with the knowledge and the tools she would need to give birth comfortably.

## Preparation for parenthood

Preparing for parenthood is essential for anyone wanting to have a baby. I think that it is even more important for couples who are struggling to have a child. I frequently work with couples who have been through years of trying but who have never thought about conceiving in terms of becoming parents. Couples sometimes become so focused on having a baby that they forget to think about anything from that point on.

The questions and approaches in this section are intended to:

- Highlight any concerns or fears they may have about parenthood.

- Increase confidence and prepare for parenthood.

- Highlight any conflicts between the couple about parenting.

- Encourage communication between partners and help them both to have more insight and understanding about how the other was raised.

- Help the couple to consider how they want to parent and what is important for them.

- Help the client to become a conscious parent, rather than someone who unconsciously repeats their parents' responses and patterns of behaviour. The way that we were parented is deeply ingrained in our unconscious mind and unless we are conscious of that we are likely to repeat our parents' parenting style, whether we like it or not.

## How can we be good parents?

Becoming a parent can seem an overwhelming and daunting prospect for some people, and they may feel that they don't know where to start. Many people have heard and seen differing and conflicting ideas about how to parent and may be confused about what is the 'right' and 'wrong' way of going about it.

Maggie Chapman, therapist and Chief Executive of META charity (Mind Education Through Awareness) talks about the three functions of being a parent: to create physical and emotion safety, to love, and to nurture. Sharing this with your client may give them a good place to start thinking about how they want to parent. They can then ask themselves, 'How can we create a safe, loving, and nurturing environment for our child?' Understanding their parental role in this way can also inform them about how they would handle day-to-day situations throughout that child's life. Essentially, if you are providing safety, love, and nourishment for your child in any given situation, you will be successfully fulfilling your role as a parent. You can encourage your clients to think and talk about how this could be applied in different situations as your child grows through life.

Ask the following questions:

- Why would a baby want to be born into your household?
- Why wouldn't a baby want to be born into your household?
- What do you trust in your partner?
- What don't you trust in your partner?
- What do you feel safe about in your relationship?
- What do you like about your present relationship with your partner?
- How do you think having a child would alter your relationship?
- What aspects of being a parent do you look forward to?
- What aspects of parenting do you think you wouldn't like?
- How adequate do you feel as a mother? (Scale 0–10)
- How confident do you feel in your ability to be a mother? (Scale 0–10)
- What do you believe needs to change for you to become a good parent?
- What kind of parents do you want to be?
- What do you believe is fundamental for a child's wellbeing?
- What are the qualities and values you want to instil in your child?
- When your child is a young adult (age 21–25), what kind of person would you like them to be?
- How are you going to help your child to become self-sufficient, emotionally secure and able to function in the world?

*Hypnotic tools*

- *Pseudo-orientation / Future Pacing*: to create a clear idea of their child as a '25-year-old' who is self-sufficient, emotionally secure and able to function in the world in a healthy way.

- Visualisation: being the parents they want to be.

- *Resource Gathering*: to access the qualities that the client feels they need to be the parent they would like to be, for example, patience.

- *Polarity Exercise*: to create acceptance of all possibilities. This is very good for those who demand perfection of themselves as a parent. Example: *I allow myself to make mistakes and get it wrong as a parent, and I very much look forward to it. I also allow myself to be a fantastic parent and do all the right things, and I very much look forward to it.*

*Self-help / Homework*

- Ask your clients to watch and observe other people and how they parent and ask themselves how they would do it differently. Ask them to discuss it with each other and find out how they would choose to do it.

- Ask your clients to think of someone whom they think is a good parent. What do they do that lets you know they are a good parent? Watch them and talk to them, in order to find out more about their attitude to parenting.

- Give your clients a few questions to go home with, that they can reflect on and discuss with their partner in between sessions:
    What are my core values? And what are yours?
    What values do we want our children to have?
    How was I raised? How were you raised?
    What do I like and dislike about how I was raised? What do you like and dislike?
    The most important thing I learnt about raising children when I was growing up was … What did you learn?
    What things have we both decided are not negotiable (for example: completing school)?

### Case study: preparing for parenthood

Annalise came to see me a few weeks before she was due to start IVF because she felt conflicted about whether or not she wanted to go ahead with it.

She had been previously married, as had her current partner. During her first marriage, soon after she had a child her husband left her. He had been unable to cope with the responsibilities of fatherhood and felt that the baby had 'ruined' their marriage.

Her current husband's previous relationship had come to an end because after his first child was born his wife had suffered severe post-natal depression and been unable to take care of the baby. He had been left with all the responsibility and had raised the child on his own.

Now, a few years later, my client recognised that both her and her husband have a number of concerns about parenthood and were equally worried that having a baby together might affect their relationship. They had not spent very much time discussing their respective concerns, although they both acknowledged feeling some ambivalence about having a baby together.

Annalise felt very confident in herself as a mother and her concern was more about how they would parent a child together. She knew that her concerns were all unfounded and were merely an 'irrational overshadow from the past'. She wanted to trust and believe that having a baby together would not ruin their relationship. I asked her how true that statement felt to her now on a scale of 0–10 where 10 represented 'completely true'. Rationally she knew it was completely true but she said that at the moment it felt about 5 out of 10. I got her to tell me all the reasons why it was a 5 rather than a 0. During this conversation she explained all the ways in which this relationship was different from the last, and told me about all the qualities that her husband had which suggested he would support her and be a good father.

In *Stage 2: Balance* I used the *Self-Integration Dissociation* to clear out the past events that were affecting her perception of the current situation. I suggested that she breathe out any old experiences that were causing her to doubt her husband and their ability to sustain a good relationship with a new baby. Once she had cleared out the overshadowing past experiences, I suggested that she breathe in the qualities she would need to be able to clearly see if and how, they could happily parent a child together. I suggested that the process that she had now started could continue in the days and weeks ahead so that she could feel more and more confident.

After the trance session I suggested that she talk to her husband and find out more about what his concerns were. I suggested that they both answer and discuss the following questions:

- Why do you want to have a baby?

- Why don't you want to have a baby?

This conversation brought things out in the open, after which he decided to work through his concerns with a therapist.

In the following session with Annalise, I used *Parts Work* to work with the part of her that still believed her husband would leave her if they had a baby together. The part presented itself as a broken egg; she said it looked fragile and devastated. Feelings of heartache and sadness moved her to tears as she saw that this part was just trying to protect her from further disappointment. She accessed a 'soothing, comforting part' that scooped up and cradled the broken egg. By holding the sadness and the heartache she was able to separate the past from the present. She imagined the egg yolk and egg white dividing up, and saw the 'soothing, comforting part' taking care of the past heartache.

Now that the disappointment was being safely held in the past, I asked her what that part was able to see about her current situation. She said that she felt as if a thick mist had lifted. I suggested that she look forward with her new found clarity and notice what she could see in her future. She smiled and said she could see a group of bright yellow baby chicks. Once she had integrated this change in perception we did a *Pseudo-orientation* so that she could see herself and her husband with a baby and notice how they were parenting the child together.

As a homework task I asked her to discuss the following with her husband:

- How would we like to parent this child?

- What is my role as a mother?

- What is your role as a father?

- How are we going to share the responsibility?

> Since both of them had experienced parenting alone, they now were able to think through what it would be like to do it together, and how they could make it work in a way so that both of them could feel supported and happy.
>
> Preparing for parenthood and addressing the fears that she had about having a baby allowed her to have/undergo the IVF treatment knowing that she was doing it because she did in fact want it to be successful.

## *Preparation for medical treatments*

Preparation for medical treatments requires a combination of knowledge about the upcoming medical treatment, access to useful inner resources and self-help tools, and an attitude of positive expectation.

An important part of preparing clients for medical treatment is ensuring that they have the resources they need to be able to deal with the outcome. If they feel equipped to be able to handle and tolerate the treatment failing they will be much more likely to feel relaxed during the treatment. For this reason, ego strengthening and resource building are key components for preparation. The following approaches are recommended:

- *Self-Integration Dissociation*
- *Resource Gathering*
- *Parts Work*
- Ego strengthening suggestions
- *Anchors.*

Most of the information about working with people who are having medical treatment can be found in *Section D: Assisted Reproductive Technology (ART)* (Page 308). There are three treatment plans for working with ART which are all designed, in part, to prepare clients mentally, emotionally and physically for medical treatment. When working with clients who are undergoing medical treatment, ask:

- If you were mentally, emotionally and physically prepared for the treatment, how would you know?

- What needs to change in order for you to feel prepared for this treatment?

- What would help you to feel more ready and prepared for this treatment?

## Stage 6: Support

The focus of Stage 6 is to support and help the client maintain some of the changes that have been made.

For one reason or another, many people feel unable to talk to family and friends about their fertility problems, and as a result their difficulties tend to leave them feeling isolated and alone. Emotional support is a basic human need that, when lacking, can result in disturbances in mental, emotional and physical health.

In this section I give suggestions about the ways in which we can offer emotional support in specific circumstances such as during pregnancy, after loss, when fertility treatment has failed, when a crucial decision needs to be made, or when it's time to move on.

Throughout the book I have suggested a variety of ways to create change. When your client has made changes to the way that they think, feel or behave, it is important to support them in maintaining these changes. This section provides tools and techniques which help clients maintain the positive changes that they have made. Relapses and setbacks are a normal part of the process of change and supporting your client through them becomes key to their ongoing transformation.

**This section contains:**
- Support to maintain change
- How to maintain change
- The importance of emotional support
- Support during pregnancy
- Support after miscarriage and stillbirth
- IVF and other medical treatment failure
- Choosing not to become parents
    - Deciding when to stop trying
    - When the decision has been made

- The effects of infertility
- Looking at the options for parenthood
- Moving on
  - Grieving, acceptance and integration
  - Finding meaning, purpose and direction.
- Working with men

## Support to maintain change

*Failure to change does not result from an inability to follow through. It most often results from an internal conflict between the desire to change and the ease of doing what you are used to doing.*
Steven Bercov, Mental Health Counsellor

Change can be uncomfortable. It often requires a deep commitment to tolerate the discomfort that may arise in the process of transformation. If people are mentally prepared for this challenge, they will be able to recognise when they are outside their comfort zone and see this as a good sign that things are changing. People will be better able to tolerate any unease if you reframe the discomfort of change in this way.

In order for change to continue it needs to be nurtured and nourished. Below is a story about the importance of daily attention and practise in order to nurture change. The story illustrates the importance of regular daily practice in order to reap the lasting benefits from a seed of change. I am particularly fond of this story for fertility clients because it can help reduce stress and worry by instilling an attitude of positive expectancy.

### A story about creating change

*I once knew a young girl who lived in the middle of the city, in a tall building on the top floor. When she was 4 years old her grandfather came to visit and brought a gift with him. The gift was a small green pot filled with soil. When he gave it to her, he told her that the gift would only truly be hers if she agreed to do as he said. She felt so excited about the mysterious pot that she promised to do anything her grandfather asked. He told her that she had to promise that every day, without fail, without exception and without excuse she would half fill a little jug, and pour the water onto the soil. But she had to promise to do it every single day. That seemed easy enough and so she quickly agreed to do as he said.*

*The next morning she woke up really early, filled with excitement, and half filled the jug and emptied the contents into the pot. The following day she did the same. A week later she began finding it harder to remember to do what she had agreed. Nonetheless she made an effort to water the pot as she had promised, even if it turned out to be late in the day. Every day she looked at the pot expectantly, wondering what the gift may be. As the days went by and there seemed to be no sign of change in the pot, she began to lose enthusiasm. So she wrote a letter to her grandfather impatient to know how long it would be before the gift revealed itself. Her grandfather replied saying that not he or anyone else could know the answer to that, and that she should continue doing as she had promised because sooner or later the gift would be revealed.*

*Determined to receive her gift she persisted day after day. And then one morning she awoke without expectation, and as she was pouring the water into the pot she looked at the soil and noticed a bright green shoot beginning to surface. With absolute amazement and wonder she realised that she had begun receiving her gift. And every day that little plant grew more and more and brought the young girl such joy and delight that watering it every day became effortless and fun. Until at last the now strong plant grew bright pink flowers that filled her bedroom with the most delightful fragrance.*

## How to maintain change

Use the following approaches to help your client to tolerate the discomfort of change and to nurture and nourish the seeds of change they have planted in their life.

Ask the unconscious

- Ask the client in trance to *become aware of what you can do on a daily basis to maintain this change in your life.*

- The ideas that arise from the client are inevitably going to be the most meaningful and effective for them.

The Fertile Body Method

Cues and reminders given as suggestions in trance.

- Cues and reminders given in trance can prompt clients to carry out a particular thought or action.

- A cue could be anything from a colour to a word or a sensation:
    - e.g. *Every time you see the colour orange you will be reminded to take a deep breath and relax your body.*
    or
    - *Each time you see a small baby you will be reminded to tell yourself that you are doing everything you can in order to create the best possible chance of conceiving.*
    or
    - *Each time you feed your cat you will be reminded to drink plenty of water throughout the day.*

*Anchors*

- *Anchors* can give the client access to a resource state which could help them tolerate the discomfort of change more easily.

*Pseudo-orientation / Mental Rehearsal*

- Pseudo-orientation in time, also known as future pacing, can be used to instil and maintain changes. It invites the client to travel in their imagination to a time in the future where they are continuing to experience the new thoughts, feelings or behaviours.

Conscious attention

- Remind your clients that the simplest way to nurture change is to give it their attention. For example: *If you are learning to be more calm and relaxed you would need to give yourself and your body regular attention so that you could know when you are no longer feeling relaxed.*

- Attention cultivates deeper awareness and helps people become more conscious of unhealthy habits and behaviours.

*Self-Hypnosis* recordings

- Recording the session and giving it to the client on a CD or MP3 so that they can listen to it on a daily basis.

- Repetition is a very effective means to create long-lasting change.

Many of the self-help tools in Section C (Page 279) provide simple activities that can be done on a regular basis to maintain and promote change. I have highlighted some particularly useful tools below.

*Self-Hypnosis*

- *Self-Hypnosis* as a self-help tool that can be used in many different ways and is an invaluable way of maintaining change.

*Affirmations*

- An affirmation is a positive statement phrased in the present tense that holds significant meaning for the person working with it e.g. *I am feeling deeply relaxed and confident in my body's ability to conceive.*

- In order for an affirmation to be effective it needs to be repeated regularly and it is important that it is not just the words that are being said, but that the feeling behind the words is being evoked and experienced. Using the above example, it is important to access a feeling of relaxation and confidence as you say these words out loud.

- *Affirmations* can be said at any time. They can also be very effective when used during *Self-Hypnosis*.

- Visualising and seeing yourself feeling deeply relaxed and confident in your body can further increase the effectiveness of the affirmation.

Keep a journal

- Keep a daily journal to note the positive changes that have occurred.

Daily exercise

- Suggest an appropriate daily exercise that can be done every day to reinforce a thought, feeling or behaviour, e.g. rub your belly to reinforce your confidence in your capacity to be pregnant; visualise yourself holding a baby in your arms; or use a daily journal to record the ongoing positive changes.

*Emotional Bank Account*

- The *Emotional Bank Account* can be checked every day so that the client can be consciously aware of whether or not they are maintaining a healthy *Emotional Bank Account*.

*Quick Body Scan*

- Scanning is a very simple and effective way of maintaining relaxation on a day-to-day basis.

## *The importance of emotional support*

Emotional support is particularly important for those who are dealing with major life challenges. For some people, having a baby is one of the most difficult life challenges they will be faced with. People who have good emotional support are likely to experience far less of the negative effects of infertility.

Firstly we need to determine whether or not the client is receiving the support they need, and then we can offer suggestions about how they may be able to get further support if needed.

*Questions*

- To what extent do you feel supported?
- Who are you able to talk to about this?
- Who do you feel really understands what you are going through?
- Do you know anyone else who has experienced something similar?

Emotional support can be provided by partners, friends, family, professionals and support groups. Dr Alice Domar strongly advocates fertility support groups in her mind-body fertility programme. Research shows that group support can help people with just about any health problem to feel better (Domar, 2002, p. 73).

An infertility support group offers compassion, friendship and understanding. Being part of a group of people who have shared a similar experience can help people recognise that their feelings are normal and natural. The group can also provide advice for coping with difficult situations, such as enduring fertility treatment. Group support is particularly useful when a difficult decision needs to be made or when coping with a loss. Please refer to Section E for some recommended support groups (Page 355).

## Support during pregnancy

Support during pregnancy is especially important when there has been a history of miscarriage, loss or birth trauma. Typically, the woman needs to build and maintain confidence in her body and to decrease anxiety and worry. The information provided in *Prepare for pregnancy* in *Stage 5: Prepare* suggests many useful techniques and self-help tools that prepare the client for pregnancy.

When the woman is actually pregnant, regular support and ongoing help can be invaluable.

*Case history / education*

- Give the couple time to talk about any concerns or fears that they have.

- Ask solution focused questions to find out how they would prefer to be thinking, feeling and behaving.

- Teach them one or two of the self-help tools below to manage their anxiety throughout the pregnancy.

- Reassure them that concern is normal.

- Suggest that they try to take one day at a time.

- It may be sensible to tell close friends and family that they are pregnant before 12 weeks, so that they can be supported by them.

*Self-help tools*

- *Mindfulness*: to stay present and take one day at a time.

- *7:11 Breathing*: to increase relaxation.

- *Nurturing*: to generate feelings of wellbeing during pregnancy.

- *Quick Body Scan*: to maintain physical relaxation during pregnancy and to notice the positive signs of pregnancy.

- *Self-Hypnosis*: to practise the *Three Steps Forward* technique or for positive mental rehearsal of pregnancy.

- *Mini-Break Anchor:* to manage anxiety or fear if it arises during the pregnancy.

- EFT: to work through any specific unhealthy thoughts or feelings about the pregnancy.

## Support after miscarriage and stillbirth

Here are some ideas about how we can support people who have recently lost a baby due to miscarriage or stillbirth. For more information about how to work with internal conflict or emotional disturbance resulting from miscarriage and loss, please refer to *Stage 3: Resolve* (Page 89).

The most important way to support people after they have experienced the loss of their baby is by witnessing, listening and allowing them to feel whatever it is they are feeling.

It can be very challenging to witness the pain and despair that your client is experiencing. But simply being present to their sadness can provide them with a safe place to grieve. Women often tell me that it is sometimes hard to talk about their loss to friends and family because they seem to feel rather uncomfortable discussing it.

Some clients need to be given permission to grieve and connect with their feelings about the loss. Since miscarriage is a fairly common occurrence, it may be handled insensitively by other professionals who could imply that an early loss is insignificant. Remind clients not to underestimate their loss, because although they may have miscarried very early on in their pregnancy, the loss still signifies the end of their baby's life.

*Case history / education*

- Suggest that they give themselves time and space to grieve.

- Recommend that they seek out support from friends, family, professionals and other women who have miscarried.

- Encourage them to talk to their doctor and wherever possible get information about the cause of the miscarriage.

- Ask them how they feel about their loss.

- Ask them how their partner is handling it.

- Find out whom they have told about their miscarriage.

- Find out what they think would be helpful for them at this time.

*Approaches*

- *Self-Integration Dissociation*: can provide a safe supportive internal space in which they can grieve.

- *Bird Cage Release*: to emotionally let go of the lost baby.

- *Grief Ceremony*: suggest that they find a way to honour their baby's memory.

- Write a letter to your baby: say how much you love them and how sorry you are that they didn't survive.

## IVF and other medical treatment failure

If possible, encourage your client to create a long-term treatment plan, so that if a treatment is unsuccessful, they have already thought about what their other options are. This can help them to keep things in perspective.

When clients know that they are about to embark on their final attempt at IVF, this can create added pressure and stress. A challenging but necessary approach to deal with this pressure is to address the possibility of the treatment being unsuccessful. If clients are able to start coming to terms with the possibility of the treatment not working, this can reduce the pressure and allow them to have a healthier attitude towards the medical treatment.

When you have been working with someone in preparation for IVF treatment, you need to be aware of the risk that the treatment will fail. We know that on average IVF results in a relatively low number of live births (for statistics please refer to *Success rates for ART,* Page 316). If treatment does fail, we need to be ready to support couples.

When clients tell me that their treatment has failed, I offer my condolences and spend some time asking them how they feel about it. Giving them an opportunity to talk about the result and the impact it is having on them, their partner and other areas of their life can provide some much-needed emotional support.

Make a note of any self-damning or self-blame as they talk about the treatment failure. It may be necessary to address unhealthy beliefs surrounding the failure of the treatment. Some typical statements that may need to be challenged include:

> *I'm obviously just too old for this to ever work.*
> *I just know that it's never going to be successful.*
> *I was very negative throughout the treatment, so it's probably my fault that it didn't work.*
> *It's impossible that I will ever actually get pregnant.*
> *I just feel so useless.*

### Case history / education

- Remind them to allow themselves to feel lousy; it is a very normal, natural response.

- Recommend that they consciously practise kindness and compassion with themselves.

- Find out what they are pleased with that they did during this IVF cycle.

- Ask what has helped them to feel better in the past when they have experienced a great loss.

- Ask them whether they know someone who has been through something similar. How did they cope? What did they do that was helpful?

- Find out if they think they may need to take a break from treatments.

- Ask what would help them recover from the treatment.

- Find out what they could do to make themselves feel better?

*Approaches*

- *Cognitive Restructuring*: to challenge any thoughts about treatment failure that are negatively affecting the way they feel, for example *'It hasn't worked and I know it's probably never going to work.'* Being conscious of this kind of thinking lets clients acknowledge that the treatment has not worked while at the same time helps them to realise that this doesn't necessarily mean that it will never work.

- *Nurturing*: self-care is a good way for clients to prevent lapsing into hopelessness, self-sabotage or feelings of worthlessness. Self-nurturing can increase feelings of wellbeing after treatment failure. It can also aid physical recovery.

- *Self-Hypnosis:* encourage your client to continue doing regular relaxation as this will help them manage the effects of an unsuccessful treatment.

- *Resource Gathering*: to access coping skills and inner resources.

- *Inner Guide*: to find out what would be most helpful for them at this time.

- *Gratitudes*: are a good way for clients to keep perspective after such a big disappointment.

- *Self-Integration Dissociation*: to develop a sense of protection from other people's comments. After treatment failure, people can feel especially vulnerable to 'good news' from friends or thoughtless comments from family members.

- *Grief Ceremony*: to process the grief and loss resulting from treatment failure.

## Choosing not to become parents

When a couple have been having problems with their fertility, unless they go on to have a baby, there will come a time when they will be faced with some important questions about when to stop trying and what to do next. In this section I address these important questions and suggest some possible approaches for supporting your client through these difficult decisions. Finally I have included some ideas about how to work with those who choose not to become parents or find they are unable to adopt.

## Deciding when to stop trying

When will you stop treatment? When will you stop trying?

There is no right answer to these questions. Knowing when to move on can be difficult. Some people have the choice taken out of their hands because they are forced to stop trying. They may have no more money to spend, or the doctors may have advised them that they have little or no chance of success. However, for those who are not forced to stop, the above question can be a very difficult one to answer.

Partners often have very different ideas about when it is time to stop. If a couple disagrees on when to stop trying, it would be beneficial for them to see a therapist together or separately to resolve the issue. If the disagreement is not addressed it may result in the breakdown of their relationship.

Clients often tell me that they feel as if their lives are 'on hold', that as long as they continue trying they feel as if their lives are slipping away 'unlived'. It may be that the couple decide that they have had enough and simply want to get on with their lives.

After numerous treatments and tests, people may get to the point where they feel they just can't handle the thought of 'anything more to do with fertility'. When they feel as if they just can't stand it anymore, they are usually ready to begin considering stopping. Although some people think that they will just go on and on with treatments until they get pregnant, they may find that their body just can't take it anymore.

On average, couples with fertility problems undergo medical treatment for three to four years. If they have not conceived after this time, they may be left feeling that they have spent a lot of time and money and have nothing to show for it. Often they say they just feel empty.

If you and your partner were to decide now to stop trying, what would that be like for you? How would you feel?

This may be the first time some people have been faced with this question, and they may be surprised to find that they feel a sense of relief at the thought.

Others experience anxiety and fear at the prospect and feel they are not ready to 'give up'.

*Questions*

- How will you know it is time to stop trying?
- If you do decide to stop, what would be the implications of your choice?
- What are the reasons you want to make this choice?
- What are the reasons you don't want to make this choice?
- What is your partner's attitude to stopping?
- How will you feel about this choice ten years from now?
- What would you like your life to be like if you don't have children?
- What are you looking forward to now?

*Approaches*

- *Inner Guide*: to seek guidance and insight about stopping treatment.
- *Parts Work*: to resolve internal conflict about making a choice.
- *Meditation*: to quieten mental chatter so that intuitive guidance can arise.
- *Out of The Box*: to get a different perspective on the situation.

# When the decision has been made

When a couple decides to stop trying they are likely to feel a mix of emotions. It is important that they recognise that stopping trying, whether it is their choice or not, marks the beginning of a new journey. Finally, after whatever they have been through, they are now faced with the reality that they will not be biological parents. Until now there has always been a glimmer of hope, but the cessation of trying marks the beginning of coming to terms with the way things are.

Grieving the loss of biological parenthood can be extremely difficult. As with all loss, it will take time to heal. There is no short cut and no quick way to make it okay. Some people may spend all their time 'wallowing' in their feelings. They become stuck and unable to move forward in their lives. Others may be quick to move on and pay little attention to how they feel about their loss. A balance between allowing the feelings and moving on is needed. Each person needs to follow their own needs and take as much time as they need to grieve.

Some people may seek out other avenues such as adoption as a way to avoid the pain and sadness that they feel. Unfortunately, nothing can heal grief except the process of grieving. In order for couples to be ready to consider other options, they need to have taken time to fully mourn their loss.

*Approaches*

These approaches can help couples to come to terms with the fact that they will never have their own biological children.

- Write a letter to their unborn child telling them how they feel about the fact that they will never meet them and know them.

- *Grief Ceremony*: have a ceremony to mark the 'end of trying' and to say goodbye to your 'unborn child'.

- *Self-Integration Dissociation*: to breathe out and let go of being a biological parent.

- *Healing White Light*: to clear and release the parts that are holding on to being a biological parent and allow the light to bring peace and acceptance.

- *Inner Emptiness Reintegration*: to create acceptance of their decision to stop trying.

- *Pseudo-orientation / Future Pacing*: to see themselves coping and living a fulfilling life without children or with adopted children.

- *Bird Cage Release*: to help them let go.

## The effects of infertility

Infertility often has a big effect on a couple's self-worth. Find out what effect their infertility has had on how they feel about themselves.

Some typical responses include:

*I'm not a real woman / man.*
*I'm a failure.*
*I'm useless.*
*I'm inadequate.*
*My body doesn't work.*

### Approaches

- *Cognitive Restructuring*: to challenge the belief *I am a failure because I have not been able to have my own biological child.*

- *Resource Gathering*: to build self-worth and self-esteem.

- *Doors Of Perception*: to see the effect that their belief is having.

- *Parts Work*: to work with the part responsible for the belief that they hold as a result of not being able to have a baby.

- EMDR: to desensitise the unhealthy belief and install a healthy belief.

- EFT: to address the unhealthy belief resulting from their experience.

## Looking at the options for parenthood

There are always other options to consider. Depending where a couple is in their fertility journey they may feel more or less ready to consider other paths to parenthood. A decision to stop trying does not necessarily mean they are choosing to be childless.

As a therapist, it can be difficult to know when the right time may be to raise these issues. For some people, discussing what they will and won't consider as options can provide a very safe context in which to pursue medical treatment. They will feel better knowing that there are many different ways to realise their dream. Others may feel that serious consideration of other options such as adoption is premature, and that they are not yet ready to 'give up hope' of having their own children.

Some people find the idea of non-biological children inconceivable and push the idea to one side without carefully considering it as a possibility. While it may be true that other paths to parenthood are not right for them, it's good to encourage your clients to explore these options with an open mind before drawing any conclusions. It can be quite a hard idea to get your head around having a child who is 'technically not your own', and yet when people start to consider the idea, learn more about it, talk about it and familiarise themselves with the possibility, they begin to feel excited about it.

If your client is thinking about, or has already decided to stop trying for a baby, ask them whether or not they have considered sperm or egg donation, surrogacy, or adoption. The aim is not to convince them of one option or another, but rather to make them aware of their options so that they can make a conscious choice.

I would recommend that they find a support group or talk to other people who have been in a similar situation and who have chosen donation, surrogacy, or adoption. Hearing other people's stories can get people thinking about these possibilities in a new way.

In cases where couples are in disagreement about sperm or egg donation or adoption, find out whether the partner who is against it has made up their mind or whether they are just not yet ready to do it. Elicit their concerns; suggest that they list all the reasons why they do not want a non-biological child. Once these have been identified you can look more closely at the reasons and work through any issues that need to be resolved or challenged.

### Approaches

- *Regression*: to explore why your client feels uncomfortable about adoption, even though they may not consciously be able to put their finger on it.

- *Parts Work*: to gain insight into the inner conflict surrounding having a non-biological child.

- *Pseudo-orientation / Future Pacing*: to see themselves with children who have been adopted, and so on.

- *Out of The Box*: to get a different perspective on a possible scenario.

*Self-help tools*

- *Self-Hypnosis*: regular relaxation is of great importance during the decision-making process. Doing *Self-Hypnosis* once or preferably twice a day will reduce emotional arousal and help the client think more clearly about their options.

- Keep a journal: suggest that they write down all the reasons why they are against having a non-biological child. These reasons can then be looked at more closely during a session.

- *Cognitive Restructuring*: to challenge some of the beliefs that have been identified to determine whether or not they are valid reasons for not wanting a non-biological child.

## Moving on

Choosing not to be parents may be one of the hardest decisions a couple has to make. Only when the decision has been made can they begin the process of moving on. But what does 'moving on' actually mean for those who have come to the end of their fertility journey?

Many of us have learnt that moving on means putting the past behind us, forgetting about it, and shutting down the way we feel about what has occurred. On some level this may seem to be the 'easiest' way of moving on. There is, however, another way of moving on, which can bring wholeness and deep healing and allow your clients to harvest the fruits of their experience.

The *Fertile Body Method* looks at two main aspects to moving on:

- Grieving, acceptance and integration.

- Finding meaning, purpose and direction.

### Grieving, acceptance and integration

Each and every experience we have in life offers us the opportunity to discover a deeper intimacy and compassion for ourselves. The gifts of our experiences are only unwrapped by our willingness to embrace and accept the entirety of what has occurred and how we feel. At the heart of this blessing is our capacity to love ourselves just as we are. To consciously move on, richer and more whole as a result of what we have experienced, is a possibility available to all of our clients.

Working towards acceptance and integration is at the core of healing. Even when the client has, to some degree, come to terms with the possibility that they may not have children, at the point at which they decide to no longer pursue it, a far deeper level of acceptance is needed. Rather than this being a passive acceptance of failure or hopelessness, or however they think of it, what is needed to truly move on is an active acceptance. Active acceptance means consciously integrating and allowing all of the different or conflicting thoughts and feelings to be a part of you. When getting clients to move on in this way, we are helping them reach a place of self-acceptance, self-love and inner peace.

*Approaches*

- *Polarity Exercise*: to create cognitive integration.

- *Self-Integration Dissociation*: to facilitate integration and self-acceptance. *'Bring in all parts of yourself, breathe in and allow yourself to include all aspects of your journey and recognise them as parts of who you are. Be curious about what it feels like to allow yourself to lovingly hold all parts of who you are.*

- *Inner Emptiness Reintegration*: to release judgement and labelling and heal their relationship with their fertility.

- EFT: to integrate and accept all parts of themselves.

- *Storm Cloud* metaphor.

- *Parts Work*: to acknowledge and integrate all parts; to find acceptance for all parts.

- *Grief Ceremony*: to acknowledge their feelings about their loss of parenthood.

## Finding meaning, purpose and direction

Along with accepting and integrating the loss and coming to terms with not having children, moving on can be facilitated by getting a sense of meaning, purpose and direction in one's life.

*Questions*

- What have you gained from this experience?

- What have you lost?

- What is the most useful thing that you have learnt?

- In what ways are you different as a result of this experience?

- If there is some 'reason' why you had to go through all of this, what do you think it might be?

- How has this affected other areas of your life (relationships/family/work etc.)?

- When you think about the way you handled and dealt with this, what are you proud of?

- What difference is this experience going to make to how you live your life from now on?

- How can this experience you have been through together become a resource for you both?

- How could you use what you have experienced to help others?

- What are you grateful for?

Ensuring that your client is having their needs met is an important part of helping them come to terms with infertility. Find out what having children would've given them. This may provide you with some information about their underlying needs, so that they can take steps to find other ways of getting those needs met.

Another important part of the process of moving on is to begin exploring the question: 'Who am I without children?'

- What do you want to do with your life?

- What are your dreams and hopes?

The Fertile Body Method

The *Creative Task* of making a collage showing 'the life that you now envisage for yourself' can be a very powerful way of helping your client to reconnect with their purpose and desires.

*Homework*

The following questions (Petty, 2005) will encourage your client to explore their purpose more deeply. Suggest that they work with these questions for a period of time each day, writing down any thoughts and ideas that arise.

1. Who am I?
2. What do I want?
3. Where do I belong?
4. What are my core needs?
5. What are my core desires?
6. What are my core beliefs?
7. Am I being true to my core beliefs?
8. What makes me happy?
9. What would I do if I had an endless supply of energy, time and money?
10. What are my main gifts and strengths?
11. Am I using my gifts and strengths to their fullest? If not, why not?
12. What are my main challenges?
13. What do I have to give others?
14. For what do I want to be remembered?
15. Have I had a positive impact on the world? If not, why not?
16. What is my legacy?
17. What would I do right now if I had a magic wand?

A copy of these questions, available on the resource CD, can be printed out and given to your client to take home and work with.

## *Working with men*

Although almost half of all known fertility problems are related to the man, in my experience they are far less likely to seek professional help, except perhaps sometimes in cases where their wife has made the initial contact. More often than not I work with just the woman which unfortunately drastically reduces the effectiveness of treatment.

One possible way of circumventing this problem is by working 'indirectly' with the man. Encourage the woman to share what she has learnt with her husband so that he too can benefit from the knowledge and tools that she finds helpful. Give homework tasks, where appropriate, that involve the husband and encourage open communication between them. This alone can sometimes have a wonderful effect on the man. Another option is to offer the man a hypnosis CD designed to address his particular problem, for example *The Big Race* visualisation for men with poor sperm mobility or the *Breathing Colour* relaxation technique to reduce stress.

Problems with sperm count and motility are particularly sensitive issues for men, and many of them feel humiliated and ashamed and believe that it reflects negatively on their manliness and power. The *Primal Image* is a very useful tool for working with sperm problems. In one case I asked a man to think about his sperm and tell me what image came to mind. He described his sperm as 'injured soldiers limping into battle' and laughed at the vivid picture in his mind's eye. I asked him to imagine how that image would need to change in order for him to know that his sperm were able to fertilise his wife's egg. He said that the soldiers would become like medieval knights, well protected and clad in armour. Each knight would be on horseback, riding into battle on a strong and fast stallion. I used this wonderful imagery to guide him into 'battle' where one special knight rescued and saved the kidnapped maiden.

Testosterone which triggers sperm production is governed by the hypothalamus-pituitary-axis which is sensitive to emotional tension. As with women, heightened anxiety and ongoing stress can reduce male fertility by negatively affecting sperm production.

When medical treatment such as IVF/ICSI needs to be pursued because of a male factor it can result in the man blaming himself and feeling guilty for what the woman has to go through. Because medical treatment is a lot harder on a woman's body, she may find that she feels resentful or angry towards her husband for having to go through it. Sometimes this is an outspoken issue, but often guilt and resentment goes unmentioned for fear that mention of it may cause major disruptions in the relationship.

In a case where the fertility problems had been a male factor, the woman confided in me saying that she really didn't want to go through another IVF cycle but her husband insisted that they just keep trying until it worked. She had tentatively mentioned the idea of sperm donation to him, and he responded to it with such anger believing that her suggestion obviously meant that she didn't want to have a baby with him after all. The conversation escalated into an argument which ended with her reassuring him that she did want to have HIS baby, and that they would just keep trying IVF until it happened. In cases such as this, couples counselling may be beneficial.

Sexual performance anxiety is a common problem which tends to affect men who feel pressurised to perform during the woman's fertile time. One of my male clients explained how he and his wife had been trying for a baby for nearly three years. As time passed his wife had become more and more desperate to have a baby and he was left feeling as if she only even 'wanted' him for a baby. Even when he had been working late and felt really tired she would insist that they have sex. As a result of this pressure he found he was unable to maintain an erection. Initially he had put it down to his tiredness but when it started to happen more and more frequently he began to worry about it. By the time he came to see me he said he had become so anxious about it that it was all he could think about when he was with his wife. He developed a fear of it happening which exacerbated his stress levels causing it to happen more frequently. In our work together we talked about how he could improve the situation with his wife. Central to our work was helping him to restore his confidence and increase relaxation. The *Polarity Exercise* helped him to cognitively shift his demand to perform and his fear of not being able to maintain an erection. He used the *Polarity Exercise* as a self-help tool to reduce his anxiety whenever he thought about having sex with his wife.

The following issues tend to affect men:

- Anxiety about medical treatments and giving sperm samples.

- The negative effects of lifestyle restrictions imposed to improve fertility.

- Sexual performance anxiety such as erectile dysfunction and premature ejaculation.

- Reduced libido.

- Concern about what other men think and upset by teasing and male bravado.

- Unhealthy beliefs about themselves as a result of poor sperm diagnosis.

- Concerns about responsibility and fatherhood.

- Relationship problems.

- Feeling unable to 'keep up' with their wife's demand for sex.

For those with concerns about fatherhood please refer to the suggestions for preparing for parenthood in *Stage 5: Prepare* as well as the *Recommended reading* in the Resources section (Page 351).

# Section C: Techniques, Scripts and Tools

The following section includes a selection of hypnotic techniques, scripts, metaphors and self-help tools. A list of the techniques and scripts can be found below and a list of the self-help tools can be found on page 279.

All of the techniques which are marked 'Can be done without formal hypnosis' do not require a traditional hypnotic induction nor do they require any knowledge of working with hypnotic phenomena. These techniques can be used as a guide for the session. Therapists should always be watching the clients and reacting 'in the moment' to the client's response as they are going through the treatment so that they can continually adapt what they are saying and how they are responding to the client's experience.

So, although many of these techniques here do not require formal hypnosis training it is necessary that inexperienced therapists receive training from a tutor, and practise it under their guidance before working with clients.

## *TECHNIQUES AND SCRIPTS*

- 7:11 Breathing .................................................................183
- 10 to 1 Self-Hypnosis .....................................................184
- Breathing Colour ............................................................186
- Safe Place/Favourite Place ............................................188
- Primal Image ..................................................................190
- Doors Of Perception ......................................................192
- Resource Gathering .......................................................194
- Self-Integration Dissociation ........................................196
- Control Room .................................................................200
- Parts Work ......................................................................202
- Rewind Technique .........................................................206
- Free Floating Regression ...............................................208
- IMR Signals – to locate past events ..............................211
- Somatic Bridge Regression ...........................................214
- Anchors ...........................................................................216
- Apposition Of Opposites ...............................................218
- Polarity Exercise ............................................................221
- Three Steps Forward .....................................................223
- Fear Release ...................................................................224
- Inner Guide ....................................................................227
- Pseudo-orientation/Future Pacing/Mental Rehearsal ....229
- Free Floating Pseudo-orientation .................................231
- Out of The Box ...............................................................233

- The Storm Cloud ................................................................. 235
- Inner Emptiness Reintegration ................................... 236
- Body Talk .......................................................................... 239
- Word Association ........................................................... 243
- Hypothalamus Meditation .......................................... 244
- Bird Cage Release ........................................................... 246
- Cellular Memory Recall ................................................ 248
- Healing White Light ..................................................... 251
- Healing Green Light ..................................................... 254
- Creating A Fertile Body ................................................ 256
- Connect With Your Inner Body ................................... 259
- Tune Into Your Body Clock ......................................... 261
- Fertility Garden .............................................................. 263
- IVF Preparation .............................................................. 264
- Embryo Transfer ............................................................. 267
- Implantation ................................................................... 270
- The Mirror Of Forgiveness .......................................... 272
- The Big Race .................................................................... 274
- Conception ....................................................................... 276

**Acknowledgement:**

The scripts and techniques included here have been contributed, influenced and inspired by a number of people over the years. I have tried to give credit where possible, but would like to apologise to all those who I have been unable to name.

## 7:11 Breathing

Can be done without formal hypnosis.

*Brief description*

The *7:11 Breathing* exercise takes its name from the length of the inhale and exhale. This technique can be demonstrated to the client by placing the palms of your hands on the diaphragm (base of your ribs) with your fingers pointing towards each other. You then breathe in for the count of seven, pause for a moment and then exhale for the count of eleven. This breathing is done in through the nose and out through the mouth. The exhale is done as if breathing out through a straw. Your shoulders should remain relaxed throughout and your hands should move apart as your ribs expand to indicate abdominal diaphragmatic breathing. The script below can be used as a guide, but the best way to teach the 7:11 is by demonstrating it to the client and getting them to practise it in front of you.

*Main aims*

- To induce relaxation – an elongated out-breath stimulates the body's natural relaxation response.
- Use as a self-help tool – it can be done as a regular relaxation exercise or used for instant relaxation in a stressful situation.

*When would you use it?*

- This should be taught to everyone who is feeling stressed or anxious unless they already have a technique they are using effectively.
- This breathing technique is particularly good for panic attacks and phobias.

*Contraindications*

- This is not suitable for people who feel more anxious when they focus on their breathing.

*Script*

> If you ever feel stressed, anxious or fearful you can use this deep breathing technique which is called the 7:11 to regain control and to induce a feeling of relaxation in your body and mind. Breathe in slowly and gently through your nose for the count of seven. Pause for a brief moment before exhaling out through your mouth for the count of 11. Continue to focus on the counting as you breathe. Repeat this until you feel calm and relaxed. You will know that you are engaged in diaphragmatic breathing if your hands move apart as you inhale.

*How can it be adapted?*

If breathing in for seven and out for the count of eleven is too difficult, it can be adapted to 3:5. The important thing is to slow the breathing down and elongate the out-breath.

*Source*
Joe Griffin and Ivan Tyrrell (Griffin and Tyrrell, 2007, p. 85–6)

---

## 10 to 1 Self-Hypnosis

*Brief description*

When the client is in a state of deep hypnotic relaxation you can then teach them this *Self-Hypnosis* technique. Include suggestions for regular practice and easy learning. Upon awakening the client, explain the steps for entering hypnosis once more. Then ask them to demonstrate it. Once they have been into and out of the trance, answer any questions they may have regarding this practice.

*Main aims*

- To induce relaxation through entering the hypnotic state.

- Self-help tool which can be used for affirmations, visualisations and other hypnotic techniques.

*When would you use it?*

- For clients who would benefit from a systematic and structured approach to entering trance.

- To teach someone the skill of *Self-Hypnosis* for affirmations, visualisations or other hypnotic homework.

*Contraindications*

- This technique is not recommended for people with low mood or depression because of the suggestions for drifting 'down' which could exacerbate symptoms.

*Script*

> I am now going to teach you self-hypnosis … you will learn … how you … all by yourself … can go into this wonderfully relaxed state … all you have to do is to … find the time and the place where you can … be comfortable … and have a reasonable chance of being undisturbed … you then make yourself comfortable … you can sit down or lie down … as long as you are comfortable … you then gently allow your eyelids to close … and with your eyes comfortably closed … you begin … silently and mentally … to count down from ten to one … you count slowly … at the same rate as you breathe out … or even at every second out-breath … that will slow you down … and with each descending number … between ten and one … you are going to become … one tenth more relaxed … ten per cent more relaxed … with each descending number … each descending number … will help you to … go one tenth deeper … into that wonderful … hypnotic state of relaxation … the light trance state … that in any event … will become deeper and deeper … as you practise … and when you reach the number one … you will be as deeply relaxed … as deeply in the trance … as you are now … in fact … you might go much deeper … because each time you practise … you become more proficient … and each time … you go deeper than before … now … when you are in this relaxed state … you can give yourself positive … beneficial suggestions … (insert relevant suggestions about how they

can use this time in trance) ... ... and you can stay in this relaxed state for as long as you like ... when you practise last thing at night ... it may even turn into natural sleep ... and to awaken from this wonderful state ... all you have to do is to ... silently ... mentally count up from one to ten ... and with each number ... you become a little more awake ... and by the count of ten ... your eyes can open ... and as soon as your eyes open ... you will be fully alert ... and each time you awaken from the trance ... you awaken feeling fine ... rested ... renewed ... rejuvenated ... you wake up feeling better ... than you have felt in a long ... long time ...

*How can it be adapted?*

- This can be adapted for people who are better able to visualise by including a pathway, set of stairs or other similar device that they see themselves moving down while counting.

*Source*
London College of Clinical Hypnosis Certificate Course

---

## Breathing Colour

Can be done without formal hypnosis.

*Brief description*

This technique combines visualisation and breathing to induce a state of deep physical relaxation.

*Main aims*

- To induce relaxation.

*When would you use it?*

- For people who are anxious about hypnosis.

- To reduce stress.

- For those who would benefit from doing *Self-Hypnosis* relaxation.

- Use this technique to precede the *Self-Integration Dissociation*.

*Script*

As you rest there, just allow yourself to become more aware of your breathing … paying special attention to the difference between your out-breath and your in-breath … notice how each time you inhale, your body is receiving everything it needs … fresh air, oxygen, nourishment … and each time you exhale … your body is releasing and letting go of everything it no longer needs … carbon dioxide and waste … and if you pay special attention to your out-breath … you'll notice that each time you exhale your body is releasing and letting go … become more relaxed with each breath.

So as you continue to breathe … easily and effortlessly … you can use your mind's eye … to scan your body … from the top of your head … down to the tips of your toes … and as you scan your body … so you can notice … any parts of your body where you are holding on to any tension … and you can be aware of that tension in the body … as a colour … so that as you scan your body … you are creating an internal map … showing you the parts of your body … that are filled with this colour …

And when you are done … you can shift your attention to the air around your body … and become aware that the air around your body … is filled with the colour of relaxation … and so each time you breathe in … you are breathing in this beautiful colour of relaxation … breathing it into your body … and each time you breathe out you are breathing out the colour of tension … breathing that tension out of your body with each breath …

And you can really use your in-breath … to breathe that colour of relaxation down to the parts of the body that need it most … breathing it deep inside … and then breathing out … and letting go … of that tension … so that slowly … breath by breath … your whole body is being filled … with that beautiful colour of relaxation …

As your body begins to feel more relaxed … you'll notice that your mind is beginning to relax too … as you allow each breath … to carry you …

to deeper and deeper relaxation … you are more and more comfortable … and that relaxation can continue to deepen … with each breath … as we go on …

*How can it be adapted?*

It can be done as *Self-Hypnosis*.

*Source*
Written by Sjanie Hugo

---

## *Safe Place / Favourite Place*

Can be done without formal hypnosis.

*Brief description*

This visualisation technique guides the client into either a 'safe place' or a 'favourite place of relaxation', depending on what is needed therapeutically. Suggestions are given to build the safety and comfort of this place, so that everything they need to feel secure and at ease is available to them. The safe/favourite place may be somewhere which they have actually been before or it may be somewhere imaginary that they create in the trance state, the important thing is that they know that nothing and no one can enter this place without their permission.

*Main aims*

- To induce deep relaxation
- To create a sense of safety
- To give the client access to needed resources
- To stabilise and build ego strength.

*When would you use it?*

Use the *Safe Place / Favourite Place* as part of *Stage 2: Balance* and specifically if you are intending on doing any *Stage 3: Resolve* work using *Regression,* EMDR or EFT. *Safe Place* can also be taught as a form of *Self-Hypnosis* and be used in preparation for medical treatment, surgery, pregnancy, birth etc.

*Script*

> Allow your eyes to close … and as soon as you do you can relax more deeply … just allow your body to make the most of this opportunity … by releasing and letting go of any tightness or tension … enjoying the relief that comes when you choose to relax … and just let your breath release all of that effort … from the past days … as you breathe out … becoming more relaxed and comfortable with each breath …
>
> As your body continues to ease out … and this relaxation begins to feel more and more pleasurable … so you can let your mind drift … let your mind go … just let it float away … like in a pleasant dream … drifting any place you choose … following thoughts of comfort and ease … just letting yourself drift and float … towards a special place … towards a place deep inside you … which is filled with long, long forgotten feelings of safety … perhaps it is a place you have been to before … or perhaps it is a place that you are discovering now … in your creative imagination … it really doesn't matter … as long as this place fills you with a sense of complete safety and peace …
>
> And as you arrive in this special place … you will notice your mind and body becoming even more restful … even more peaceful … because you know that in this place … nothing can bother you at all … in this place you are surrounded by all the things that you love … and you can notice these things around you now … bringing such a deep sense of comfort … in this special place which is so perfect for you at this time … everything is just right … the temperature … the light … the aromas … all fill you with an ever-deepening sense of relaxation and calm …
>
> In this retreat … this oasis … this paradise … everything feels good … to the touch … to the skin … as if you were lovingly wrapped in comfort … and you can just notice how much you really can enjoy this place … doing whatever feels good … knowing that in this place you are totally free … to be who you are … and enjoy that freedom in whatever way

you choose … because this place is just for you … and for no one else … almost as if it has a strong impenetrable boundary around it … so that nothing can enter without your permission …

And as you continue to enjoy the peace, freedom and safety of this place … so you can feel your whole system becoming ever more deeply relaxed … as you absorb and receive all the benefits that being in this special place brings … receiving all the goodness, the pleasure … the comfort … letting it sink deep inside your mind and body … so that this feeling of safety can stay with you … this feeling of comfort can be kept deep inside … your special place … always inside … knowing you can return here whenever you choose … benefitting deeply now from just being in this place … helping you to feel so much better in the days ahead … just relaxing and absorbing all that this place gives …

*Source*
Written by Sjanie Hugo

---

## *Primal Image*

Can be done without formal hypnosis.

*Brief description*

A primal image is a symbol which arises from the unconscious mind which represents our current beliefs, perceptions and physiological state. A primal image can be elicited for just about any different aspect of fertility, e.g. reproductive system, womb, sperm, birth. This image can then be worked with to restore wellbeing and enhance fertility. It is easier and more effective to work with one aspect of fertility at a time.

*Main aims*

- To get insight into beliefs, perceptions and physiology.
- To influence the mind and body positively.

# Techniques, Scripts and Tools

*When would you use it?*

Use the *Primal Image* during *Stage 1: Outcome* as a tool for goal setting, or in *Stage 4: Enhance* to work with physical problems and enhance fertility.

*Script*

Step 1: Elicit the image through questioning

> **As you think about your** (reproductive system, womb, ovaries, sperm, penis, or sexual relationship) **now, what image comes to mind?**

Step 2: Create change

> If you knew you were in a healthy fertile state, how would that image be different?
>
> or
>
> How does that image change when your body is in a healthy fertile state?
>
> or
>
> If you were a baby about to be conceived, would you consider that womb to be a safe, nourishing and loving place?
>
> or
>
> As you think about being a healthy sexual and sensual being, how does that image change?
>
> or
>
> *Imagine you are an artist with all the tools and colours you may need at your disposal. Using these tools, and colours, what changes would you like to make to this image in order to make it safer? More nourishing? More fertile? More sensual? More welcoming? More loving? More* (client's words)?

Step 3: Integrate change

> When all the necessary changes have been made to the image, suggest that the client sees this image being reabsorbed back into the appropriate place in their body.
>
> Suggest that they consider what differences these changes will have on them in their day-to-day life. Ask them to imagine themselves at a time in the not-too-distant future behaving differently, thinking differently and feeling different as a result of these inner changes which they have made.

*Source*
Inspired by Maggie Chapman
Written by Sjanie Hugo

---

## *Doors Of Perception*

Can be done without formal hypnosis.

*Brief description*

The *Doors Of Perception* is a visualisation that allows the client to experience the effects that a particular unhealthy belief is having on them both now and in the future. It also allows them to experience the benefits of a new, healthy belief. Once they have experienced both 'doors' they are given an opportunity to choose which door they would like to go through and how they would like to continue living their life.

*Main aims*

- Change limiting beliefs
- Instil a healthy affirmation
- To come to terms with possible outcomes.

*When would you use it?*

In *Stage 2: Balance* this can be used to challenge and change unhealthy beliefs. It can also be used to assist resolution and decision making in *Stage 3: Resolve* or *Stage 6: Support* by testing two alternative outcomes or choices and the benefits and effects of each.

*Contraindications*

Depression could contraindicate the use of this for future outcomes, since it may prevent the client from being able to access a healthy and happy future.

*Script*

- Imagine that you are standing on the pathway of your life
- As you stand on the pathway of your life, look ahead and notice that the path forks and along each path there is a doorway
- Your life continues beyond both of those doorways
- Through the first doorway, you will continue living your life with the belief _____ (the client's unhealthy belief)
- Through the second doorway, you will continue living your life having chosen to believe _____ (the client's healthy belief)
- When you are ready, go through the first doorway
- As soon as you are through the door, you become aware that you believe _____ (unhealthy belief)
- You can continue living your life with this belief, and notice how you feel … notice how you behave … become aware of how your body feels … as you continue to believe that
- Become aware of how this belief affects your work … your relationships … your friendships … your health … and your fertility …
- PAUSE
- Now, return to the path
- When you are ready, go through the second doorway
- As soon as you are through the door, you become aware that you believe _____ (healthy belief)
- You can continue living your life with this belief, and notice how you feel … notice how you behave … become aware of how your body feels … as you continue to believe that

- Become aware of how this belief affects your work … your relationships … your friendships … your health … and your fertility …
- PAUSE
- Now, return to the path
- In a few moments you are going to wake up, but before you do, you can make a choice, and decide which doorway you are going to walk through
- So that as soon as you are fully wide awake, you can live your life with that belief, with those feelings, and with those outcomes
- When you have made your choice, please let me know
- (Awaken)

*Source*
Inspired by Avy Joseph
Written by Sjanie Hugo

---

## *Resource Gathering*

Can be done without formal hypnosis.

*Brief description*

*Resource Gathering* takes the client back to a time in the past when they have experienced a particular resource that they would like more of in their current or future situation. When the client is recalling this past experience as if it were happening now, the therapist suggests that they allow the positive feelings to grow. As soon as they are fully experiencing the positive resource state, they hold onto the feelings and bring them into the present. They can then see themselves in a future situation thinking and behaving in the way they would like to, as they continue to experience the resource state.

*Main aims*

- Build resources
- Build ego strength
- Prepare for future situations.

*When would you use it?*

- In *Stage 2: Balance* to restore balance when a particular resource is needed to restore balance.

- To access resources needed to solve problems and meet challenges.

- To build self-esteem.

- To help stabilise and strengthen prior to doing any work in the *Stage 3: Resolve*.

*Contraindications*

Depression may contraindicate the use of this technique since the client may find it difficult to access positive past memories and recall resource states.

*Script*

- (Identify the resource that is needed before starting the trance session)
- Recall a past time when you have experienced _____(resource)
- Experience it fully using all of your senses
- Imagine the intensity of this experience growing so that you are experiencing _____(resource) more strongly
- Notice the changes in your body as _____(resource) becomes stronger
- Continue experiencing _____(resource) as you return your awareness back to the present
- Still deeply connected to this _____(resource), see the events of your life as a landscape across time
- Notice how this _____(resource) changes your perspective of upcoming events
- Notice how this _____(resource) can be used to resolve some of the difficulties that you have been having
- Zooming in on a particular future event, notice how you respond differently
- Notice the positive effects that this _____(resource) is having on the way you think, feel and behave … notice how it is changing your perception of this experience in a positive way

*How can it be adapted?*

Resources can also be gathered by imagining being a person, real or imaginary, who has the inner resource that the client needs.

They can also be taken forward to a time when they have resolved the difficulty to become aware of what they have done in order to create the change, and then to bring that resource back with them to the present.

*Source*
Inspired by Robert Dilts (Dilts, 1980)
Based on the work of Milton H. Erickson, M.D.

---

## *Self-Integration Dissociation*

Can be done without formal hypnosis.

*Brief description*

This visualisation uses the concept of a mental and emotional boundary combined with breathing to create a safe, protected inner world which is clear from any obstructions/disturbances which may be affecting the goal.

*Main aims*

- To create a sense of safety and protection.
- To develop strong emotional boundaries.
- To change a belief or behaviour.
- To clear and release beliefs, emotions, behaviours or past experiences that may be negatively impacting on the goal.
- To receive the needed resources, learnings, perceptions and behaviours.

*When would you use it?*

During *Stage 2: Balance* to create balance and increased ego strength. In *Stage 3: Resolve* it can be used as an indirect or metaphorical approach for resolving issues. In *Stage 5: Prepare* it can help clients prepare mentally and emotionally for an upcoming event such as IVF, pregnancy, birth or parenthood.

*Script*

> You can be aware of your whole body, particularly the skin that surrounds your body. Notice how your skin very clearly defines your physical boundary. Your skin very clearly separates everything that is you from everything that is not you. And the wonderful things about your skin, is that it is strong and flexible, too. Your physical boundary is strong enough to keep all of you safely inside, and it is flexible enough to allow you to move and grow. And I'm sure you are aware that your skin is permeable, which means that your body is able to release things through that boundary, such as sweat, waste and impurities. It is also able to absorb things into the body that the body needs, such as moisture, sunlight, and warmth.
>
> In just the same way as your body has a physical boundary, you have a mental and emotional boundary. Your mental and emotional boundary very clearly defines everything that is you from everything that is not you; it contains all parts of you. And just like your skin, this boundary is strong and flexible. It is strong enough to protect you and keep you safe, and it is flexible enough to allow you to grow, learn and evolve. Your boundary has an opening that can be sealed shut whenever you choose. And through this opening you are able to release things that no longer serve you, things that disturb your inner world, or limit your full potential. You can release any psychological and emotional waste or limiting beliefs through that opening. You can also receive and absorb what you need through that opening. You can receive new beliefs, healthy emotions, new ways of thinking, and new ways of responding, useful resources and skills. You can even receive a new way of seeing things that will allow you to recall past experiences with new perspectives.
>
> In this trance state you can become more aware of your mental and emotional boundary, you can get a clearer sense of what your mental and emotional boundary is like. Notice what size and shape it is. Become

aware of its texture; notice what it is made of. Perhaps you can see its colours, or hear its vibration. It really doesn't matter how you experience it. Just allow yourself to become more aware of it, in whatever way is right for you. You can also get a sense of where the opening is located and how you can seal it shut whenever you need to.

As you continue to breathe in and out, just notice which parts of your boundary need to be strengthened or reinforced or rebuilt. You can use your in-breath, now, to restore and strengthen your boundary. Just focus on each in-breath and allow each in-breath to help rebuild, reinforce and strengthen your mental and emotional boundary.

Take as many breaths as you need to, and when your boundary is fully restored and strengthened and in optimum condition, you can let me know.

(Wait for confirmation)
Good. With your boundary repaired and strengthened now, notice the wonderful feeling of safety and security that you are experiencing. Your strong, secure boundary is creating a shield of protection all around you, so that nothing will bother you in quite the same way.

As you continue to enjoy this ever-deepening sense of safety and security, so you can feel more and more calm and relaxed. So calm and relaxed that you become aware of your own inner world, more aware of everything that is contained within your boundary.

And as you think about _____ (insert goal, for example: being a confident mother), just start to notice anything that is inside this boundary that is preventing you from fully realising your potential to _____ (insert goal).

You can become aware of these things in whatever way is right for you. There is no need for you to consciously know what these things are. Your unconscious mind can allow you to be aware of them symbolically, as objects, colours, words, feelings or images. It really doesn't matter how you become aware of these things, the important thing is just to notice them now.

And when you are ready to move more fully _____ (for example: into becoming a confident mother) you can focus on your out-breath. Just allow each out-breath to help you breathe those things out through that opening. Notice how each time you exhale you are able to let go of those blocks and limitations. With each breath watch them move out through that opening. Feel and sense yourself releasing and clearing those old ways of being, becoming lighter and clearer with each out-breath.

When you have breathed out everything that is preventing you from realising your goal, just let me know.

(Wait for confirmation)
Good. And now that you have released those limitations you can feel yourself moving into _____ (insert goal, for example: a more confident state as a mother). Now if there is anything you need to help you fully realise your potential _____ (for example: to be a confident mother), you can allow yourself to receive that through the opening of your boundary. You may need to breathe in the feeling of _____ (mention an emotion that is relevant, for example: confidence) or the belief _____ (name the healthy belief that is relevant, for example: I can be a good mother, and I can raise a well-balanced child) or a behaviour that tells you _____ (for example: you are much more confident in yourself as a mother).

You can also breathe in some of the qualities that you feel you need more of to be _____ (for example: confident in yourself as a mother such as patience or courage). Breathe in every example you have witnessed in your life of _____ (for example: confident mothering). And as you continue to inhale everything you need, you may start to see an image of yourself _____ (for example: as a confident mother) being received through that opening. Whether you see it, sense it or just allow yourself to acknowledge it, I want you to know that your unconscious mind now knows that you are _____ (for example: so much more confident in yourself and your ability to be a mother).

When you have breathed in everything you need to allow you to be _____ (for example: confident) just let me know.

(Wait for confirmation)
Good. Now you can allow that opening to seal shut, keeping all of this safe inside. And as you continue to breathe in and out, you are allowing all of this to settle. Everything you have received can find its natural place within your inner world, just letting it all settle in an effective and harmonious way. Allow all of this to sink deep inside your unconscious mind, deep into every cell in your body. Letting it all sink in so that you

can start to live your potential as a _____ (for example: mother) in every moment and in every way.

And this process that you have started today will continue all the while you breathe. With every breath that you take, you are learning and growing and developing more and more, helping you to _____ (for example: become more confident) every day. This will continue with every breath that you take, throughout the day and even at night while you are sleeping, all the while that you breathe …

*Source*
Written by Sjanie Hugo

---

## Control Room

Can be done without formal hypnosis.

*Brief description*

This is a metaphorical mind-body approach that can be used to address both psychological symptoms (e.g. anxiety) and physiological symptoms (e.g. PMS or low sperm count). The client is guided into a control room that houses all the controls for the systems of the mind and body. Changes can be made to the necessary controls in order to restore balance and wellbeing.

*Main aims*

- To restore mental, emotional and physical balance
- To address/reduce symptoms
- To increase wellbeing
- To return a sense of control.

*When would you use it?*

In *Stage 2: Balance* to address any physical imbalances such as high FSH levels, low sperm count, irregular cycles, and so on. It can also be used to restore emotional balance and wellbeing. During medical treatments such as IVF, it can be used to improve the effectiveness of medication and to decrease some of the negative side effects.

*Script*

- Become aware of a path ahead of you. As you walk along the path, you may feel a sense of growing curiosity and intrigue as you wonder where this path leads to.
- You can let your curiosity guide you further along the path, and as you walk you can feel yourself becoming more relaxed with each step, following the path as it winds and meanders, taking you deeper into your inner world.
- Enjoying the rhythm of your walk, enjoying the sensation of the earth under your feet, breathing deeply and enjoying the fresh air, as you become more deeply relaxed with each step.
- Continue following the path until you see a doorway ahead of you.
- Reach the door and notice that it has your name on it.
- In your pocket you find the key that unlocks the door.
- Unlock the door, and enter the room.
- This is the control room of your mind-body which houses all of the controls that govern how your mind and body function.
- Take a moment to look around. See, sense and feel the magnificence of this place. Notice all the different dials, knobs, levers, buttons and controls.
- Everything is so well organised and arranged, with labels and signs so that you immediately know what each control is for.
- As you continue to explore your control room, you will soon notice the controls that are responsible for _____ (for example, reproductive system or emotional responses).
- Notice the current settings.
- Each control has an optimal setting that will restore balance and wellbeing.
- If the controls need to be adjusted to their optimum setting, you can do that now.
- Perhaps they need to be turned up or down, on or off, higher or lower. Do whatever you need to do to ensure they are at their optimal setting.
- As you make these adjustments you may notice a change or shift in the way you feel; you may notice a chemical response in your body as balance is restored. When you have finished making these adjustments, look round the control room, and notice if there are any other

adjustments to the other systems that you need to make, so that you will improve your health and wellbeing.
- (Ask for confirmation when they are done, and then lead them out of the control room. Suggest that they can return whenever they need to.)
- And as you walk back along the path, you can be curious about what changes you will notice in your day-to-day life, a result of the changes that you have made.

*Source*
London College of Clinical Hynopsis Diploma Course

---

## *Parts Work*

Can be done without formal hypnosis.

*Brief description*

*Parts Work* is based on the concept that there are many different parts to each person which together make up the whole person. The technique identifies the part that is responsible for a particular belief, feeling or behaviour that appears to be in conflict with the client's goal. While the client is in a state of inner absorption they are asked to become aware of this part of themselves and allow an image or symbol to form in their mind's eye that best represents this part. This part image is then invited to come and rest in the palm of their hand. The therapist then facilitates a dialogue with this part to elicit the part's positive intention, and negotiate a change that will support this part's intention *and* the client's goal. Other parts and resources can be drawn upon to assist in creating the change. Once the part has agreed to change and is in alignment with the client's goal, the part is then re-integrated. Once it's been fully re-integrated, the client is invited to see the positive consequences and outcomes of this change using direct suggestion and *Pseudo-orientation*.

*Main aims*

- To gain insight and understanding
- To resolve inner conflict
- To create internal harmony and co-operation
- To build resources.

## Techniques, Scripts and Tools

*When would you use it?*

*Parts Work* can be used in *Stage 2: Balance* to work with unhealthy beliefs, change bad habits and build resources and in *Stage 3: Resolve* to identify and work with unresolved issues.

*General Parts Work script*

- Access the part responsible for the belief, feeling, or behaviour
  Allow yourself to become aware of the part responsible for _____.
  Let this part come more fully into your awareness.

- Become aware of this part as an image
  And as you become more aware of this part, notice what image / symbol / shape comes into your mind to represent this part of you.

- Imagine placing this part / image into the palm of your hand
  You can imagine this part floating out and coming to rest in the palm of your hand … so that you can be aware of it, over there.

- Ask this part if it is willing to communicate
  And now, you can communicate silently and mentally with that part, aware of it in the palm of your hand, you can talk directly to it, and it can respond to you through thoughts, ideas, images, sensations and sounds. I'd like you to ask this part if it would be willing to communicate with you now.

- If the part is willing, thank the part. If the part is not willing, find out what it needs in order to be able to communicate.

- Find the part's positive intention
  Every part of you has a positive intention and is trying to do something for you. Allow yourself to become aware of this part's positive intention for you.

- Negotiate the change
  The negotiation can take any form. Essentially you are facilitating a negotiation between the client and the part that will allow the part to continue to fulfil its positive intention without the negative effects. For example:

- Thank that part for protecting you so well, and then ask the part if it would be willing to find another way to protect you that would allow you to _____ (insert the goal). Are there any skills or resources that the part needs in order to make this change now? Any others?

- Reintegrate the changed part
- Now that the part has made these changes, notice how it looks and feels different. Allow yourself to welcome that part back inside. Just imagine it floating back inside, becoming a part of you, sense and feel the positive effect it is having on other parts of you, as a harmonious balance is found between every part allowing you to fully move towards _____ (insert the goal).

- Pseudo-orientation to see the changes
- Now that every part of you is in harmony and alignment with _____ (insert the goal), just allow yourself to imagine what difference you will notice in the days, weeks and months ahead. Be curious about what changes you will notice, see yourself in these future days, doing things differently as a result of these deep and lasting changes that you have made.

*Specific Parts Work script*

This *Parts* script can be used in *Stage 3: Resolve* to help identify and address any inner conflict about having a baby.

> We are all made of different parts. Sometimes parts of us can be in conflict about what we want for one reason or another. At times we may be consciously aware of this inner conflict and other times it may be unconscious.
>
> I'd like you to hold in your mind now your intention and desire to have a baby. Let yourself feel and experience that desire in its purest, truest form.
>
> As you do that, I want you to scan your body and notice any feelings of unease or disturbance that come up. Any part of you that is not in alignment and harmony with your intention to have a baby can make itself known to you by gently creating a slight feeling of unease.
>
> Continue to observe your physical sensations and feelings, and when you are ready, let me know what you are experiencing.

(If the client describes some uneasy sensations in the body, continue. If they are unaware of anything this may indicate that there is no conflict, or that another approach may be needed.)

Are you consciously aware of what is creating this unease?

(If they are aware, invite them to share that with you, and then continue to negotiate the change that is needed.)

(If they are not aware of what is creating the conflict.) Ask your unconscious mind to make the part that is in conflict more visible to you now by allowing an image to form in your mind that represents that part of you.

What does that image look like?

What does that image tell you?

How would that image need to change in order for this part of you to be in harmony and alignment with your intention?

- Do you need to access any inner resources to make that change now? (If yes, then help them to access the needed resourse.)

Allow that part to transform now, and feel that disturbance clearing as your system comes into alignment now. Feel your mind, heart and body become more at ease and more fertile as those changes happen.

You can be curious about how these changes will show themselves to you in the days and weeks ahead.

*How can it be adapted?*

- The general script can be adapted as a resource gathering and ego strengthening technique. In this case you would be working with the resource part or accessing strengths that can be shared and developed.

- *Parts Work* has been used in many different forms and with a wide variety of conditions. There are many books available that offer a variety of examples and ways in which this technique can be adapted.

*Source*
This is a 'traditional' technique, based in part on Gestalt Therapy, and partly on the NLP technique of Six Step Reframing (See Bandler and Grinder, 1979) and the work of Roy Hunter (Hunter, 2005).

---

## *Rewind Technique*

Can be done without formal hypnosis.

*Brief description*

The *Rewind Technique* is a visual-kinaesthetic dissociation that asks the client to watch their disturbing experience in fast forward on a TV screen. Once they have played it through they are asked to step into the memory and rewind it to the beginning. This process is repeated a few times until the emotional arousal triggered by the traumatic/disturbing event is reduced.

Before beginning the process, if they haven't already done so, ask the client to tell you a bit about their disturbing experience. There is no need for them to describe it in graphic detail; however it is important that it triggers some of the disturbing response as this activates the emotional content/template connected to the memory.

Ask them to think about their experience as if it were a movie, with a beginning, middle and an end. The movie should start before there is any notion of the trauma to follow, and the end point should be a moment when they knew they had survived and made it through the experience. Make a note of the start and end point so that you can refer to them in the process.

In order for this technique to be truly effective it is imperative that the emotions related to the event are activated to some extent before you process them. This *Rewind Technique* relies on the client achieving a state of relaxation so that during the trance they can view the past experience without the intense emotional arousal.

*Main aims*

- To turn a traumatic memory into an ordinary memory

- To reduce the current negative effects of a past experience
- To resolve a past trauma or past disturbing event
- To resolve a phobic response.

*When would you use it?*

Use in *Stage 3: Resolve* for panic attacks, phobias, traumas or any past event that is negatively impacting on the person now.

*Contraindications*

- Those who are unable to relax for any reason.

*Script*

Induce deep relaxation and lead your client to their *Favourite Place*.

- Imagine that there is a portable TV screen, remote control and DVD player into which you insert a DVD of that past experience.
- Before you turn on the TV imagine floating out of your body so that you can see yourself sitting in front of the TV watching the screen.
- When you have a sense of that let me know.
- Watch yourself watch that DVD now from beginning to end in fast forward.
- When you have watched yourself finish watching it, let me know.
- Now imagine floating back into your body and then floating into that memory on the TV screen.
- Float into the end point where you know that you have survived that experience.
- In a few moments I'm going to ask you to imagine rewinding that whole experience, running the movie backwards very rapidly … all the people will walk backwards … with all the action happening in reverse … just like rewinding a movie … except that you will be inside the movie … and you will be moving backwards …
- When you are ready, begin and let me know when you are done.
- Good, now return to sitting in front of that TV screen with the remote in your hand and when you are ready, push the fast forward button and watch those images flicking past on the screen from the beginning right

- to the end of that movie, pushing pause when you have reached the end and then letting me know.
- Good, now float into the TV screen and into the end point of that movie and rewind the whole experience, running it backwards very rapidly … you're moving backwards … all the action is happening in reverse … rewinding that movie … and when you are back at the start, let me know.

REPEAT the above two paragraphs four or five times. You can then ask the client if they think they need to do it again. Repeat as many times as needed.

Use future pacing so that they can see themselves in a future time responding in a way that tells them they are free from the negative effects of the experience.

Re-orientate the client fully by asking them to return from their *Favourite Place* in the way that they arrived.

*Source*
There are many different versions and names for this technique, the original which was derived from Milton Erickson's work. An account is also given in Bandler and Grinder, 1979. This version is a considerably refined version (Griffin and Tyrrell, 2004, p. 284–9) developed by Joe Griffin and Ivan Tyrrell, co-founders of the Human Givens Approach. It is taught at MindFields College (http://www.mindfields.org.uk/) on the 'Fast Phobia and Trauma Cure' workshop.

## *Free Floating Regression*

*Brief description*

*Free Floating Regression* uses the therapeutic goal to identify a past event that may be unresolved and may be negatively affecting the client's desired outcome. Ask the unconscious mind if it is safe and appropriate to go back to a past event that is negatively affecting the goal. When the event has been identified, it can be reframed and the new learning can be re-integrated.

*Main aims*

- To identify a past event that may have a bearing on the goal
- To resolve and reframe a past event
- To integrate a new belief and positive learning.

*When would you use it?*

Use in *Stage 3: Resolve* in cases where the client is unable to consciously identify the cause of their internal conflict or resistance to achieve their goal or where a past event is negatively affecting their current situation.

*Contraindications*

- Do not use without creating safety first (such as *Safe Place*).
- Do not use if the client is lacking in internal resources and stability.
- Do not use without the client's permission.
- Ensure that you also get unconscious agreement (e.g. using IMRs).
- This approach is contraindicated for use with someone who has a traumatic past.

*Script / outline*

Induce trance.

Set up safety.

Safety can be created using the *Safe Place* script or by suggesting that the client connects with the inner resources and guidance that they will need to allow them to safely resolve whatever needs to be resolved.

Ask the unconscious mind if it is safe and appropriate to identify and revisit a time in the past which is negatively affecting the goal.

Regress.

> In a few moments time … I am going to say the word … PAST … I will repeat the word PAST … six times … and each time I repeat the word PAST … so the years are slipping away … you are drifting back into the PAST … you are drifting back to the most significant time in your PAST … when something happened to you … that not only affected you at the time … but has continued to affect you … and is continuing to prevent you from realising your goal _____ (state the goal, for example: to be a confident mother).

Repeat the above paragraph, and then say the word 'PAST' slowly six times.

> And a soon as you are recalling this event you can let me know (using *IMR Signals* or head nods).

Reframe.

Reframing can be done after hearing the client describe the event, or it could be done content free.

Possible ways of reframing the past event include:

- Draw on the resources of their 'adult self' for a new perspective
- Suggested reframes from the therapist
- Desensitise the experience using the *Rewind Technique*
- 'Re-experience' the event in a new way during trance
- Help the regressed client to access a needed resource
- Find a more appropriate way to respond to the situation, and so on.

Install new learning and belief.

Suggest that they take the learning from the experience and that they integrate this new perspective.

Positively affect all future times.

Before re-orientation suggest that all future events from this time on can be positively affected by the new learning and perspective.

Re-orientate.

> In a few moment's time … I am going to say the word … PRESENT … I will repeat the word PRESENT … six times … and each time I repeat the word PRESENT … so you are moving forward in time … you are floating forward into the PRESENT TIME (name the time, day and date) … you are returning back to the PRESENT moment … bringing all of your learning with you … so that when you arrive back fully in the PRESENT moment … you will have full access to the insights and understanding … in a way that will best help you to move freely towards _____ (e.g. becoming a confident mother).

REPEAT twice and then say the word 'PRESENT' slowly six times.

Reintegrate.

Once the client is fully re-orientated suggest that they consider how this resolution is going to positively influence the way that they think, feel and behave in future times. Encourage them to be curious about how their conscious and unconscious learning will help them move positively towards their goal in the days, weeks and months ahead.

Awaken.

*Source*
London College of Clinical Hypnosis Diploma Course

## IMR Signals – to locate past events

*Brief description*

IMRs are used to communicate with the unconscious mind to find out if there is a past event that is responsible for a current condition. If an event is identified, conscious or unconscious resolution of that event is facilitated. Once the client has been future paced to see the changes that will result, they are re-oriented back into the present.

*Main aims*

- To identify and resolve a past event that may be affecting the client now.
- To create conscious or unconscious resolution of an emotional issue.

*When would you use it?*

This technique can be used during *Stage 3: Resolve* to identify and resolve past events that may currently be affecting the client.

*Contraindications*

This approach should only be used with the client's conscious and unconscious permission. Always precede it with *Stage 2: Balance* stabilisation, strengthening and resource building. Possible contraindications include past trauma and/or abuse.

*Script*

Install IMR.

> Is there a mental or emotional cause for the problems you have been having conceiving?

IF YES: * Is it safe and appropriate for you to become aware of this cause now?

IF YES Go to A: if NO Go to B.

> **A**
> I'd like to ask your unconscious mind to let you become aware of that now, and as soon as you are, you can let me know.

Does your unconscious mind know of some past event that may have caused this mental or emotional block to conception?

Is there an earlier event that may be the cause of this block?

Let the unconscious part of your mind go back to the first event that created this mental or emotional block to conception. Review what is happening at that time, when you know what it is, your YES finger will lift. And as your YES finger lifts, so you can know what is causing your inability to conceive.

Is it all right for you to tell me about it now?

Now that you are aware of these things can you be free to conceive?

Is there anything else we need to know before you can be free to conceive?

Pseudo-orientation to time in the future when these changes will be showing themselves. For example pregnancy, birth and parenthood.

**B**
That's fine. There is no need for you to become consciously aware of that now.

Does your unconscious mind know of some past event which may have caused this mental or emotional block to conception?

You don't need to be consciously aware of any of this.

Is your unconscious mind now willing to review and resolve that past event?

IF YES: Your inner mind can resolve that event now, with all of your inner adult wisdom, letting your conscious mind have whatever insights it needs so that event is no longer a factor affecting your fertility.

When that is done you can let me know with a YES.

Are you now free to conceive?

IF NO: Ask the question below followed by *

IF YES: Continue with Pseudo-orientation

> Is there anything else we need to know before you can be free to conceive?

Pseudo-orientation to a time in the future when these changes will be showing themselves. For example pregnancy, birth and parenthood.

Re-orientate back into the present.

*How can it be adapted?*

*IMR Signals* can be used in a variety of different ways. This particular approach can be adapted to find the source of a particular belief, behaviour or physical symptom.

*Source*
Concept taken from D. Corydon Hammond (Hammond, 1990)

## Somatic Bridge Regression

*Brief description*

The *Somatic Bridge Regression* uses an emotional response to direct the unconscious mind to the origins of that learnt response. Once the emotion has been identified, the therapist suggests that the unconscious mind can find an earlier event during which the client experienced the emotional response. One or many events may be identified, creating a bridge back to the original event during which the response was learnt. Once the initiating event has been identified, the therapist reframes the client's experience so that a new, more appropriate response can be generated.

*Main aims*

- To find the origin of an emotional response.

- To resolve the original event to create a new response.

*Contraindications*

Ensure the client is fully stabilised and has good ego strength as this approach may elicit intense emotion.

*Script*

Get permission.

> Is it okay for us to explore and understand what originally happened to cause this feeling?
>
> Okay. In a few moments I will count down from five to one and as I am counting so your unconscious mind will take you back in time to a time in your recent life when you have felt that feeling of _____ (for example, anger). Focus on that feeling of _____ now as I count and your unconscious mind takes you back to a recent time when that _____ is strong. Five, four, three, two, one. Be there now.
>
> What is happening? Where are you?
>
> How are you feeling?
>
> Are these feelings new or familiar?

(If they are familiar, it indicates that there is an earlier initiating event.)

> And as you focus on these feeling now, they can form a bridge, that you can use to travel back into your past, like a road made from that feeling, allowing you to travel back further, to the origins of that feeling.
>
> *Focus on those feelings now. In a moment I am going to count from five down to one and your unconscious mind will take you back to an earlier time (perhaps the very first event that has everything to do with those feelings), a time that has everything to do with your _____ feelings. Five, four, three, two, one. Be there now.
>
> What is happening? Where are you?

> How are you feeling?
>
> Do you make any decisions at that time?
>
> Are these feelings new or familiar?

(If they are familiar, it indicates that there is an earlier initiating event.)

(Repeat the above from: *Focus on those feelings now... ) This needs to be repeated until the client reports that these feelings are new, which indicates that they are recalling the initiating event.

(If the feelings are new, use techniques to reframe the initial event. For example, bring in their adult self to offer advice, insight, support and help or to rewrite the scene.)

Re-orientate back to the present.

> And as I count from one to five, return to the present moment. As you come back to the present moment your unconscious mind is rewriting each of those subsequent events from a new perspective, allowing you to feel differently, to feel better, to think differently about yourself and your fertility ... one, two, three, four, five ... back in the present moment.
>
> Allowing all of these changes to be a part of you, a part of your inner world.

Pseudo-orientation to see the effects of the changes on future events.

*Source*
Concept taken from Lynsi Eastburn (Eastburn, 2006)

---

## *Anchors*

Can be done without formal hypnosis.

*Brief description*

An *Anchor* is a stimulus that initiates a conditioned response. Therapeutic anchors give people access to useful resources by anchoring a positive past experience. The resource state can be anchored to any cue, such as squeezing the thumb and forefinger together, that the client can conveniently and efficiently activate at the required time.

*Main aims*

- To access and develop inner resources.

- To establish a self-help tool that will give the client access to a resource state whenever they need it.

*When would you use it?*

- In *Stage 2: Balance* to develop resources and coping abilities.

- For a client who is facing difficult or challenging upcoming events, such as IVF.

*Contraindications*

Ensure that the client has had past experience of the needed resource state.

*Script*

- Agree the anchor, for example squeezing the thumb and forefinger together.
- Ask the patient to identify the required positive state (e.g. confidence or relaxation).
- Ask them to close their eyes and then go back in their mind to a time when they have previously experienced this.
- Suggest that they trigger the anchor (for example: squeeze their thumb and forefinger together) as soon as they are fully re-experiencing the feeling/state. Notice the changes in their posture, breathing, colouring and expression.

- Ask them to open their eyes.
- Repeat the preceding three steps at least four times.
- Test the anchor before the client leaves by asking them to trigger the anchor and notice what they experience.
- Encourage them to use the anchor frequently over the following few days as this will help strengthen and reinforce it.

*How can it be adapted?*

There are many different ways of setting anchors and using them therapeutically. To learn more about anchors, I recommend further study in Neuro Linguistic Programming.

*Source*
Concept taken from Robert Dilts (Dilts, 1980)

---

## *Apposition Of Opposites*

Can be done without formal hypnosis.

*Brief description*

*Apposition Of Opposites* uses the hands to restore balance to the mind and body. The client is asked to sit with their palms facing upwards so that the imbalance which they are aware of can be placed into the palm of one of their hands. The therapist suggests that they can experience the weight of that imbalance in that hand. They are then asked to imagine the opposite of that weight being placed into the palm of the other hand. Suggestions are then given to explore and experiment with how they can restore balance to their hands. Once balance has been restored to the hands the change is then integrated into the whole body and the mind.

*Main aims*

- To balance the systems of the body for fertility
- Hormonal balance

- To balance emotional responses
- To balance limiting or utopian beliefs.

*When would you use it?*

Use this in *Stage 2: Balance* to create mental and emotional balance or in *Stage 4: Enhance* as an approach to improve physical wellbeing and to enhance fertility.

*Script*

> Ask your client to sit with their hands resting on their lap, palms facing upwards.
>
> As you relax deeply now … you can start to become more aware of your body … and the many different systems that make up your body … become aware of these many different systems … such as the immune system … endocrine system and nervous system … each of these systems is made up of a variety of subsystems … and all of these systems are interconnected … and you can recognise that there is a natural and effective balance … between all the different systems of your body.
>
> Explore how you can become aware of these different systems now … It could be a physiological experience of them … or a creative, symbolic image of them … perhaps creating a mental map in your mind's eye … that represents the different systems of your body … all interconnected … all working together …
>
> Pause
>
> And now, you can become aware of the system that now most needs balancing as you work towards _____ (insert the client's goal).
>
> As you become more aware of the imbalance in that system … you can start to imagine … placing the weight of that imbalance into the palm of one of your hands … feel and experience the appropriate weight of that imbalance … in that hand … experience it in a way that's safe for you right now …
>
> Pause

And as you allow yourself to experience the weight in the one hand, you can become aware of the opposite of that weight, the lightness ... and experience the opposite in the other hand ... allow yourself to fully experience that lightness there in that hand.

Pause

Just be aware now of the difference between those hands ... perhaps you can imagine or see the difference between those hands represented by a set of scales ...

Pause

And I wonder if you know ... that one of your body's strongest drives ... is to heal itself ... is to return balance to the systems of the body ... and you can begin to engage with that potential now ... as you allow your body to return to its natural state ... allowing balance to return to those hands ... as your work towards _____ (insert the client's goal).

And I don't know if ... both hands will become heavier ... or both lighter ... one hand heavier ... or one hand lighter ... perhaps something can be added to one side ...or removed from the other ... allowing whatever change needs to happen ... so that balance can return ... to those hands ... to that system ... as you engage with your body's natural intelligence ... its powerful capacity to heal and rebalance ...

And I wonder what thought ... response ... or chemical change needs to happen right now ... in order for you to experience that balance returning ...

Pause, until balance has been restored.

And as you find that balance, allow every cell to know what that change is. And I wonder how you will begin to experience this balance right now, as it is communicated to every cell in your body?

And with that balance restored ... you can begin to wonder ... what will that new balance mean to you ... how will your life be different ... how will you experience that change ... as you work towards _____ (insert the client's goal).

(Repeat for any other systems that need to be balanced.)

*How can it be adapted?*

This can be adapted to balance thoughts or feelings instead of body systems.

*Source*
Adapted from London College of Clinical Hypnosis Practitioner Course
Inspired by Maggie Chapman

---

## *Polarity Exercise*

Can be done without formal hypnosis.

*Brief description*

The *Polarity Exercise* addresses the fears and unhealthy beliefs that create anxiety. In this exercise the client is asked to voice the demand that they are making on themselves alongside the – often unconscious – fear that has created the demand. Voicing the extremes of the 'best case' and 'worst case' scenario out loud often collapses the anxiety and re-centres the client.

The polarity statements can be repeated as homework before or during the problem situations. The client will have more control and conscious choice over their responses once they have brought their unconscious fears into awareness during challenging situations.

*Main aims*

- To create cognitive acceptance of all possibilities.
- To reduce the anxiety associated with demanding a particular outcome.

*When would you use it?*

Use this with someone who has been experiencing high levels of anxiety as a result of a limiting/unhealthy beliefs. It may be useful in *Stage 2: Balance* to create mental balance or in *Stage 3: Resolve* to resolve a belief that may be affecting the therapeutic goal. In *Stage 5: Prepare* it can be used to help the client prepare for a future situation which they feel anxious about.

*Script*

Create a scale.

> As you think about that _____ (problem situation, e.g. becoming a father) now … how do you feel on a scale of 0–10, where 10 represents _____ (goal state) and 0 represents _____ (the worst you could ever feel about it).
>
> I would like you to repeat the following statements after me … this is not an affirmation … they are just two statements that I would like you to say out loud … what you are saying might sound silly or crazy … you don't need to believe them or take them too seriously … just say the words after me …

I allow myself to be _____ (state the demand that they are making on themselves) and I very much look forward to it. For example:
I allow myself to be perfect and get everything right and be the most amazing father … and I very much look forward to it … (client repeats this statement)

I allow myself to be _____ (state the fear/opposite of their demand) and I very much look forward to it. For example:
I also allow myself to make mistakes, to get it completely wrong, and have no idea what I am doing … and I very much look forward to it … (client repeats this statement)

(Repeat these two opposing statements three times.)

Check Scale.

> Now I'd like you to think about becoming a father and let me know how you feel as you think about it now.

You can suggest that before they go into the problem situation they can say these opposing statements to themselves a few times. For example, if there is a specific situation that triggers their anxiety about fatherhood, such as being around nephews/nieces, they can say the two opposing statements to collapse the anxiety response.

*Source*
Gosia Gorna, Transformational Coach (www.gosiagorna.com)

---

## *Three Steps Forward*

Can be done without formal hypnosis.

*Brief description*

This is a guided visualisation during which the client is asked to become aware of their fears and then imagine moving them to one side where they are disintegrated or destroyed. They then take three steps forward after which they are asked to imagine an image of themselves responding in the way that they would like to.

This script is written for someone who has previously miscarried and is anxious about a repeated miscarriage; although it can be adapted and used to work with any fear.

*Main aims*

- To release fear
- To reduce anxiety
- To reinforce the goal state.

*When would you use it?*

Use with someone who is experiencing high levels of anxiety as a result of a previous miscarriage. It may be useful in *Stage 2: Balance*, to create mental balance and emotional balance or in *Stage 3: Resolve* to release the fear which may be affecting the therapeutic goal.

The Fertile Body Method

*Script*

Induce relaxation
Become aware of the fear

> Become aware of the image connected with your fear ... notice any thoughts and sensations associated with that image ...

Move it and disintegrate it

> Push the image to the left ... and imagine it being destroyed and disintegrated ... perhaps getting burnt by fire ... and washed away by water ... PAUSE ... when it has been washed away ... take a deep breath in and out ...

Move forward

> Imagine yourself taking three steps forward ...

Become aware of the goal state

> From the right ... see an image of yourself ... going through a thriving, healthy pregnancy ... notice the thoughts and sensations connected with this image ... *PAUSE* ... take a deep breath in and out ... (Re-orientate)

*Source*
Julia Indichova ('3 Steps Forward', 2002) from *The Fertile Heart® Imagery* CD

---

## Fear Release

Can be done without formal hypnosis.

*Brief description*

This script is an example of a metaphoric approach to release fear. The client is guided to imagine their book of life, which contains all of the events that have happened in their life so far, as well as the emotions which are still connected to the events. Without needing to look at them they are asked to tear out all the pages containing the fear which is preventing them from realising their goal.

*Main aims*

- To release fears that are preventing them from reaching their goal.
- Indirectly release conscious and unconscious fears.

*When would you use it?*

This can be used in *Stage 3: Resolve* as an indirect approach to resolving fears that may be preventing the client from reaching their goal for therapy.

*Contraindications*

- Fear is a survival response which is vital and necessary for healthy functioning. This approach is not intended to 'get rid of all of our fear' but rather to release the fears which do not serve us and limit our potential and happiness.
- This metaphor is contraindicated for people who hate tearing books.

*Script*

> And as you feel yourself relaxing more deeply … so you can journey in your creative imagination … letting yourself travel now … to that special place inside yourself … that safe and sacred place … that stores and holds your book of life …
>
> Your unique book of life … may be kept in a safe … or inside a cupboard … perhaps it is stored behind a glass cabinet or in a precious box … kept somewhere safe where you can easily access it …
>
> And when you reach that place where your book of life is stored … take it out … and take some time to just hold the book in your hands … feel the weight of it … notice what it looks like … and how it feels …

And as you hold the book ... take a moment to honour and respect the life you have lived ... holding the book between your hands ... as you acknowledge the life you have lived ... the events you have experienced ... the things you have learnt ...

All of your life ... is contained within these pages ... every moment of your life ... is stored away here ... in words ... in images ... thoughts ... feelings ... every day recorded and stored ...

And the wonderful thing about this book ... is that it too is alive ... it too is changing ... as you grow ... as you change ... as you perceive things differently... so you are rewriting your history ... so you are re-colouring your past ...

As you open the book now ... know that there is no need to look at the details of the pages ... but instead you can let your fingers flick through the pages ... and as you touch a page that contains an experience ... or a feeling of fear ... the kind of experience or feeling which is preventing you from _____ (insert goal, e.g. looking forward to giving birth to your baby) ... so you can loosen those pages which contain the fear ... while that feeling of fear may have been necessary at the time ... there is no need to hold onto that feeling anymore ... that experience is over ... and so you are free ... to pull out that fear now ... pulling it out ... tearing out only the unhelpful parts of those experiences ... stripping your book of dead weight ... erasing the unhelpful learning ... releasing the old stories and experiences ... which no longer serve you ... watching those pages fall away ...

There is no need to be aware of the details of the pages ... just trust your fingers ... just let yourself tear, rip and loosen ... all of the old fear ... all of the stuff that's blocking you ... that's holding you back ... that's preventing you from _____ (insert goal).

Take as much time as you need ... to reshape your book of life ... to recreate your book of life ... so that it no longer contains that unnecessary fear ... so that it no longer carries those stories filled with fear ... so that you can move forward freely ... towards a new chapter ... a new story ... that allows you to _____ (insert goal).

And when you are done ... please let me know.

Wait for head nod.

That's it … good … notice how your book of life has changed and evolved through this process … feel your book of life … new … fresh … clean … and when you are ready … you can turn to the next blank page … to a new start … and know that on these and future pages … you have already begun … living your life … without this unnecessary fear … living your life in a way that allows you to _____ (insert goal).

Return the book to the place where it is kept.

Re-orientate with appropriate ego strengthening suggestions.

*Source*
Written by Sjanie Hugo

---

## *Inner Guide*

Can be done without formal hypnosis.

*Brief description*

This is a visualisation during which the client meets their inner guide. The therapist facilitates the meeting as the client asks questions, seeks advice and receives the help they need from their guide. Before the client leaves, the guide gives the client a gift that will provide them with a needed resource.

*Main aims*

- To enable the client to connect to their inner wisdom
- To access inner resources
- To gain insight and understanding.

# The Fertile Body Method

*When would you use it?*

In *Stage 2: Balance* the advisor/guide can provide any needed resources. During *Stage 3: Resolve* this approach can be used to resolve problems and get advice, or when the client is having difficulty making a decision. In *Stage 6: Support* it can be used to provide inner support as well as maintain changes.

*Script*

- Guide the client to their *Favourite Place*.
- Ask them to invite their inner guide into their *Favourite Place*.
- Suggest to the client that they welcome their guide in and ask them to make themselves comfortable.
- Explain to the guide that they would like to gain more understanding about the symptoms they have been experiencing.

or

- Explain that they have some questions to which they would like an answer.
- The questions can be guided by the therapist or asked silently by the client.
- Suggest that they can ask the guide for whatever help or support they need.
- Allow time for this questioning process to occur.
- The guide then gives the client a gift (resource or quality). You may or may not be aware of the power of that gift, but you accept it, and thank your guide.
- Suggest that the client thanks their guide.
- Before awakening ask them to: take a few moments ... to allow the wisdom and guidance that you have received to sink in ... so that it can benefit you in the best possible way ... and as you allow it to sink in ... you can begin to imagine how this experience will benefit you ... in the days, weeks and months ahead ... you may also become curious about how the gift that you have received will be helpful to you ...
- Pause.
- Re-orientate and awaken.

*How can it be adapted?*

The *Inner Guide* can be adapted to suit the client's belief system; for example the guide could be referred to as 'a wise old person' or 'an advisor' or 'an animal helper'. This technique can also be altered so that the client imagines going inside their womb where they meet the guardian and protector of their womb; for example it could be 'a fertility goddess' or 'a fertility nurse'.

*Source*
Written by Sjanie Hugo

---

## *Pseudo-orientation / Future Pacing / Mental Rehearsal*

Can be done without formal hypnosis.

*Brief description*

*Pseudo-orientation* is also known as *Future Pacing* or *Mental Rehearsal*. During this process the client is guided to imagine their goal/future situation using all of their senses. First they are asked to observe it as if they were watching themselves from the outside and then they are asked to imagine stepping into the situation so that they can experience all the thoughts, feelings and sensations that accompany the change they want. Once the client is experiencing the future situation the therapist should always talk to them in the present tense as if what they are experiencing is happening now.

*Main aims*

- To instil new behaviour and responses.

- Create unconscious change to ensure that the client's desired behaviour and responses will occur naturally in future situations.

- To develop coping strategies for future situations.

- To rehearse new behaviours.

- To create positive expectations of themselves.

- To prepare mentally, emotionally and physically for an upcoming event.

- To help maintain healthy changes.

*When would you use it?*

This approach can be used in *Stage 1: Outcome* to get more clarity about the outcome the client wants and to reinforce the goal state. It can be used in *Stage 2: Balance* as a stabilising or resource building tool. It can also be used in *Stage 4: Enhance* to increase fertility and in *Stage 5: Prepare* to prepare for future situations. I recommend using some form of *Pseudo-orientation* at the end of each trance session.

*Script*

- Ask the client to identify their hopes, wishes and intentions for the future.
- If appropriate ask them to recall a past time in which they experienced _____ (the quality, feeling or behaviour) that they would like to experience in the future.
- Ask them to imagine that they are travelling forward in time. This can be done as the therapist counts or using a metaphorical device such as 'turning the pages of a calendar'.
- Tell them that they can travel forward to a time in the future when they will be experiencing their goal.
- Ask them to: notice what the first thing is that you will see, hear or sense in that future situation that will tell you that _____ (insert goal, for example: you are feeling more relaxed).
- First they can imagine watching themselves in this future time and suggest that they observe and notice the changes in their posture and behaviour. Perhaps they can notice how they look different, sound different and move differently.
- Then ask them to imagine stepping into the scene so that they can feel, sense and fully experience those changes. Ask them to notice how they are thinking, feeling and behaving.
- As they are doing this, the therapist can include suggestions from the outcome which has been discussed, for example: notice how much clearer your mind is … how much lighter you feel … because you are really looking forward to your baby's birth … you can feel that excitement … like beautiful butterflies in your tummy … and overall you just feel more confident … in yourself … and in your body too …
- Remind them that as they experience these changes, their unconscious mind is learning and gathering all that they need to allow them to move towards this moment in a future time easily and effortlessly.

- Re-orientate back into the present. Using the same method as was used to future orientate them (e.g. counting or the pages of a calendar).
- Before awakening suggest: your mind and body ... your whole system has now experienced _____ (goal) ... and every part of you now knows how to experience _____ (goal) ... which is why you will notice that you begin to respond _____ (for example; with confidence) in _____ (describe the future situation).
- Ensure the client is fully present by telling them the current day, date and time.
- Awaken.

*Source*
Concept taken from D. Corydon Hammond (Hammond, 1990) and Joe Dispenza (Dispenza, 2007)

---

## *Free Floating Pseudo-orientation*

*Brief description*

This is a formal hypnotic pseudo-orientation that uses the cue word 'future' to orientate the client into a future in which they can experience a time when their problem is no longer occurring. *IMR Signals* are used to communicate with the client in trance. When the client is experiencing the future situation, suggestions are made to get them to notice and learn how their problem has changed and what that is like for them. The cue word 'present' is then used to re-orientate the client back into the present moment with suggestions that they will bring whatever learning they need with them.

*Main aims*

- To help the client experience what their life will be like when the problem is not occurring. This information can be used to help create their goal for therapy.
- To access resources and learning from their 'future self'.

# The Fertile Body Method

*When would you use it?*

In *Stage 1: Outcome* this could be used with anyone who is struggling to get to grips with the change that they want. Experiencing future situations in this way may also be useful for resource gathering in *Stage 2: Balance*. It can also be used in *Stage 5: Prepare* to prepare the client for a future event as it allows them to experience the event without being affected by past problems or unhealthy beliefs.

*Script*

> Install IMR.
>
> In a few seconds time ... I will say the word ... FUTURE ... and then ... I will repeat the word ... FUTURE ... five more times ... making a total of six times in all ... now when I say the word ... FUTURE ... in a few seconds time ... and each time I repeat the word FUTURE ... so with tremendous speed ... time is rushing forward ... you are speeding forward ... into the FUTURE ... you are speeding forward to a time in your FUTURE ... when something will have happened inside of you ... that will have solved ... many of the difficulties you have been having in the past ... and as soon as you are there ... experiencing that time in the future .... when these difficulties have been resolved ... then ... and only then ... will the first finger of your right hand ... lift ... easily and effortlessly.
>
> So ready ... FUTURE ... FUTURE ... FUTURE ... FUTURE ... FUTURE ... FUTURE
>
> The pause between each FUTURE should be between 10 to 20 seconds. After the sixth FUTURE, remain completely silent. Wait for the finger to lift. (You may have to wait up to five minutes for finger movement.)
>
> When the finger goes down, proceed:
>
> That's good. And you can continue to experience your life now ... with those old difficulties resolved. Notice how you are thinking, how you are feeling ... and how you are behaving differently.
>
> Insert some of the suggestions from the information gathered pre-trance.

And as you continue to experience that more and more fully … just be curious about what else you notice is different now … perhaps you can even be aware of some of the small steps you took to get here … or possibly you may even notice how you made this change …

When you have experienced everything you need to … and you have taken all the unconscious learnings that are needed from this time … let me know by lifting that finger …

That's fine … all that you have learnt and experience can stay with … consciously or unconsciously … retaining all the learning and benefit that you have received … and in a few seconds' time … I am saying the word … PRESENT … and … when I say the word … PRESENT … in a few seconds time … you are back here with me in the PRESENT … you are back here with me in the PRESENT … and the time is _____ on _____ here _____ and you are staying completely relaxed … and you remain deeply in the trance … … so ready … PRESENT … PRESENT … PRESENT … and you are back here with me in the PRESENT … and the time is _____ on _____ here _____ and you are staying completely relaxed.

Every part of you is back here with me in the present.

Awaken.

*Source*
London College of Clinical Hypnosis Diploma Course

## *Out Of The Box*

Can be done without formal hypnosis.

*Brief description*

*Out Of The Box* uses a past spiritual experience as a resource state to help the client to resolve a problem situation.

The Fertile Body Method

*Main aims*

- To create a change in perception.

- To get more perspective on a particular situation.

- To access spiritual resources to help the client experience a situation differently.

- To gain insight and understanding about a current situation.

*When would you use it?*

Use this approach when a client feels stuck in a particular problem or when they need to change the way they are viewing a particular situation. It can be good to use with those who have been experiencing fertility problems for some time to help them regain perspective on their situation. It can be used in *Stage 2: Balance* as a resource building tool or in *Stage 3: Resolve* to help resolve a problem.

*Contraindications*

This approach would be contraindicated for someone who does not have a spiritual belief system. It can, however, be adapted by using a time in the past when they have felt deeply connected to nature, for example.

*Script*

- Access the problem state
  Just allow the problem that you have been having to come to mind and let yourself experience the effect that it is having on you ... mentally, emotionally and physically.

- Break the state
  That's fine ... you can now let your mind go blank.

- Access the resource state
  Now recall a time in the past when you felt deeply connected with something much bigger than yourself ... perhaps a moment of spiritual illumination ... or a time when you felt at one with all of life around

you … perhaps you experienced complete peace … or love … or connection …

- When the client has accessed the resource state you could ask some of the following questions:
  Where are you? What are you doing? What does it feel like? How are you thinking? How are you relating to others / environment?

- Ask the client to view the problem from this state
  Allow that spiritual moment to be present with your current problem and notice how are feeling, thinking, relating and behaving in that expansive and spiritual space … How is this different now? In what ways has the problem changed? What else needs to happen?

*Source*
Concept taken from Bill O'Hanlon and based on the work of Warren Berland (Berland, 1998)

## *The Storm Cloud*

Can be done without formal hypnosis.

*Brief description*

A metaphorical approach that uses storm clouds to illustrate nature's inevitable capacity for change and the importance of 'bad' weather for growth. This version of the script is written for 'sadness' which can be replaced and adapted to suit the client's current experience.

*Main aims*

- To illustrate the cyclical nature of menstruation
- To get clients to feel more comfortable with change
- To encourage acceptance
- To remind people that 'this too shall pass'.

*When would you use it?*

This can be used if a client feels as if their fertility problems are never going to end, or if they are going through a period of anger, sadness or pain. It can also be used in *Stage 3: Resolve* to help women understand their own cyclical nature and to restore menstrual health. In *Stage 6: Support* it can be used to help people grieve, accept their loss and move on.

*Script*

> And do you wonder … as you look down at the earth … and all that grows in it … how growth comes about? … yes … as you look down … you can realise that what you stand on is the foundation for fertile growth … but to find out what helps things grow, you need to … look upwards … look up towards the sky … a sky will change from day to day … even hour to hour … minute to minute … sometimes it is a deep and comforting blue … with the sun shining brightly … sometimes it is hazy … with clouds just drifting through … and sometimes it is dark … heavy with storm clouds … black and heavy and sad … swollen with rain … and I'm sure that you know … that growth occurs when there is rain … so even though we may not like the black … heavy … sad storm clouds … we know they are important … and there always comes a time when these clouds … release the rain … release the sadness … let the rain pour down … let it fall onto the earth … feeding … fertilising … releasing potential for new growth … and as the rain falls … so those dark … heavy clouds … become lighter and lighter … the sadness fading … as they become lighter and lighter … until the sadness … and darkness … just fade away … the sadness and darkness just fade away … and of course … it is only natural that … after the rain comes sunshine … after the rain comes blue sky … after the rain comes healthy new growth.

*Source*
London College of Clinical Hypnosis Diploma Course

## *Inner Emptiness Reintegration*

Can be done without formal hypnosis.

*Brief description*

This technique can help the client heal their relationship to their 'symptom' by disintegrating their labeling and judgement of the 'symptom'. The *Inner Emptiness Reintegration* is derived from Robert Anton Wilson's *Quantum Psychology* and is based on the concept that, on a fundamental level, everything is composed of energy.

*Main aims*

- Change the client's perception of their problem and their relationship to it.
- To reduce identification with labels such as 'infertile' or 'impotent'.
- To create peace and acceptance.

*When would you use it?*

This can be used in *Stage 6: Support* to help those who are struggling to find acceptance of their situation. In *Stage 3: Resolve* it can be used to help people resolve some of difficulties they are having regarding their situation.

*Script*

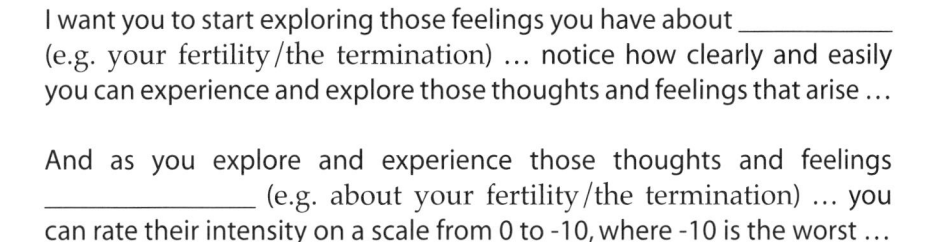

> I want you to start exploring those feelings you have about _____ (e.g. your fertility/the termination) … notice how clearly and easily you can experience and explore those thoughts and feelings that arise …
>
> And as you explore and experience those thoughts and feelings _____ (e.g. about your fertility/the termination) … you can rate their intensity on a scale from 0 to -10, where -10 is the worst …
>
> What number are you on that scale now?

Okay, that's fine ... now notice the sensations in your body ... notice any sensations in your body that accompany those thoughts and feelings that you have about _____ ... and I wonder if you can create an image ... in a way that is appropriate for you ... create an image that fully represents those thoughts ... and feelings ... and bodily sensations ...

That's fine ... and I would just like you to notice that it is you who is observing this image that represents those thoughts ... and feelings ... and now ... I want you to do an interesting thing ... I want you to look below the surface of this image ... by tearing back the surface layer ... and I want you to become aware of what is hidden underneath ...

Encourage the client to verbalise their experience.

And you can tell me what you find ...

Suggest that your client continues tearing back the layers as they talk about their experience at each stage. This should continue until they report 'nothingness', or an 'emptiness' that has no emotional content. Then suggest that they can take some time to enjoy the peace, safety and tranquility within this inner emptiness.

And as you enjoy that peace ... and tranquility ... I want you to look up above yourself ... and to notice those layers ... that you have stripped away ... notice those layers just drifting and floating in this emptiness ...

And now ... I would like you to imagine ... or experience in your own way ... those layers ... as a swirling mass of energy ... perhaps noticing the colour ... the texture ... perhaps even noticing any sounds that accompany them ... experiencing this swirling mass of energy in your own way ... a way that is appropriate for you ...

And I want you to notice too, how ... that space ... that emptiness ... that surrounds that swirling mass of energy ... is made of the same substance as that mass of energy ...

And now ... I want you to imagine that every other thought ... and feeling ... in your mind and body is made of this same substance ... no dividing lines ... just everything made of an inner energy ...

And now ... I want you to imagine that every part of your mind ... and physical body ... is made of the same natural energy ... no dividing lines ... everything made of this energy ...

And now … in a strange and interesting way … I want you to imagine … just imagine that everything around you is made of the same natural energy, too … no dividing lines … just everything made of energy … everything in this room … the chair … the walls … the floor … myself … even the air around you … everything made of this same natural energy …

As you continue to imagine … I want you to imagine that … everything outside this room … everything in (name the town or city you are in) … is made of this energy … the people … the buildings … the vehicles … the roads … the plants … all made of this swirling mass of natural energy …

And so … your imagination can expand … and you can imagine everything in this country … the towns … the cities … all made of this swirling mass of natural energy … that continues to expand … no dividing lines … one mass of natural energy … as you imagine everything on this planet made out of this energy … the countries … the seas … the atmosphere … all made out of this swirling … natural energy …

And now … imagine the entire universe … and imagine that it, too, is made of the same energy … natural … swirling energy … the planets … the moons … the stars … all made out of energy … no dividing lines … the same natural energy …

PAUSE

That's it … and now … become aware of _____ (e.g. your fertility / the termination) and notice what you experience …

Notice what number the intensity of your feelings are now on that scale …

(The intensity should by now have reduced.)

*Source*
Based on the work of Stephen Wolinsky (Wolinsky, 1991) and Robert Anton Wilson (Wilson, 1990)

## Body Talk

Can be done without formal hypnosis

*Brief description*

This script can be used to communicate with any part of the body that your client wishes to understand more deeply. It can be particularly useful for physical conditions which have a harmful effect on fertility, such as fibroids, endometriosis or poor sperm morphology. If a part of the body that needs to be visited for a particular symptom is unknown, suggest that your client scans their body to notice the place that is calling for their attention as they think about their problem.

Always let the client interpret the experience. Sometimes the meaning of an image may not be clear right away so suggest that the client keeps revisiting the body part during *Self-Hypnosis* until the meaning becomes clearer.

The script below is written for someone with fibroids and should be adapted to suit the symptoms or problems you are working with.

*Main aims*

- To understand any emotional factors that may be causing or contributing to a physical symptom.
- To determine what changes will benefit the client's condition.

*Script*

> And I know that you know ... that your body communicates with you all the time ... like when you feel a sensation in your bladder that tells you it's time to go to the toilet ... or when you feel a fullness after eating that tells you it's time to stop ... or like the physical tiredness you feel before sleep ...
>
> Your body is your ally ... your oldest friend and your steadiest companion ... it is a storehouse for your experience and wisdom ... often wiser and more attuned to your life than your mind could ever know or say ...

Techniques, Scripts and Tools

and it's always striving to work with you … to maintain balance in your system …

One of the strongest drives within your body … is a drive to heal itself … and when your body needs your support and help … it sends you messages … about what is needed when …

Sometimes we are aware of what our bodies are telling us … and often we are too busy thinking … or doing … to notice our body's messages … and sometimes all we really need … is to listen closely … to understand what our body is trying to say …

And as you continue to relax deeply … I want you to know that in this hypnotic state of relaxation … you can start to become more sensitive to your body … and you can start to sense what it is trying to tell you … through those symptoms you have been experiencing …

And now … just imagine that the fibroid is pulling you into your body … is drawing all of your attention and awareness into your body … feel that fibroid drawing you down into your uterus … and your awareness can be like a tiny camera … a small powerful camera that is able to see and sense … that fibroid … there in your uterus …

And as you go inside your body … you will become more aware of that fibroid … because you are paying such close attention now … and listening so closely to the sensations … your body can let you feel that fibroid in the gentlest way … just enough so that you can be aware of it … and you can be aware of that fibroid in the way that is best for you right now … perhaps imagining what it looks like …

PAUSE

As that mental picture becomes clearer in your mind, so the fibroid is communicating with you … through impressions and feelings … through thoughts and ideas … all of your inner senses opening up … to receive these messages … this wisdom …

PAUSE

As you listen … and sense the fibroid's message to you … you can start to see what you can do differently … so that your body no longer needs to send those signals …

PAUSE

The therapist can now ask the client to verbalise what they are aware of and what messages they have received. Ask the following questions so that the client can make the changes they would like to make.

- Are there any resources or tools you will need to do this?

- Do you feel ready, willing and able to make these changes now?

- (If Yes) You can now promise your body that you will _____ (the promise).

Notice how pleased your body is ... let yourself see how this change is going to positively impact the other systems and organs in your body ... `perhaps you can even see yourself in the not too distant future ... blossoming with fertility and new life ...

And finally ... take some time now ... to thank your body ... for everything it does for you ... let yourself feel the gratitude that you have for your body ...

PAUSE

And you can continue to listen to your body ... more and more in the days and weeks ahead ... because you know that being in touch with your body ... means you'll become more in touch with who you are ...

*How can it be adapted?*

Other useful questions that your clients can ask their body in trance:

- What was going on in my life when these symptoms first started?

- If this _____ (e.g. fibroid) could speak, what would it say?

- What do I need to know about what I am experiencing?

- Why am I experiencing these symptoms now?

- What am I doing to make these symptoms worse?

- What can I do to improve them?
- What changes can I make?

*Source*
Written by Sjanie Hugo

---

## *Word Association*

Can be done without formal hypnosis.

*Brief description*

In a waking state or a light trance state the therapist asks the client to say all the things that they associate with a particular word, for example 'fertility' or 'menstruation'. The therapist makes a note of the client's associations.

*Main aims*

- To make the client become aware of their conscious and unconscious associations with the word.
- To make a note of the client's abstract and metaphorical associations that can be used therapeutically in future sessions.

*When would you use it?*

Use this to help clients become more aware of their unconscious associations with specific words and concepts. This can be a good technique to use in *Stage 1: Outcome*, to clarify the goal. If, for example, the client's goal is to be in an optimum state to conceive, you could do the *Word Association* with them to identify how they perceive 'fertile'. It could also be used in *Stage 3: Resolve* to help identify any blocks to conceiving, for example, you could ask for their associations with 'baby' or 'parenthood'.

The Fertile Body Method

*Script*

> In a few moments I am going to say a word to you ... and without thinking about it ... I would like you to say out loud ... all the things that you associate with this word ... just say whatever comes into your mind ... there is no right or wrong ... just say as many things as come to mind ...
>
> So ready ... _____ (insert the word).
>
> Repeat with any other relevant words.

*Source*
Concept taken from psychoanalysis
Written by Sjanie Hugo

---

## Hypothalamus Meditation

Can be done without formal hypnosis.

*Brief description*

The following guided imagery is based on a script written by hypnotherapist James Schwartz. It can help to enhance fertility by addressing the effects of stress on the hypothalamus.

The hypothalamus is a small gland located at the base of the brain that communicates with the pituitary gland to control the flow of hormones in the body. Emotional responses such as stress can affect the functioning of the hypothalamus causing a disruption to the production of LH (luteinising hormone) and FSH (follicle stimulating hormone) by the pituitary gland. The hypothalamus acts as a control centre in the brain for reproductive activity.

*Main aims*

- To reduce stress
- To create hormonal balance
- To regulate hormones such as LH and FSH.

*When would you use it?*

Use during *Stage 2: Balance* to restore balance to the mind and body. Use in *Stage 4: Enhance* to address any hormonal imbalances which are affecting fertility.

*Script*

> Imagine that you are stepping into a small room. As you enter the room you notice that there is a red button on the wall with the letter S on it. When you are ready you can press that button, and as soon as you do so you will become very small, just like Alice in Wonderland. As soon as you are ready, press the button and imagine yourself becoming smaller and smaller. When your size has reduced significantly, look around and you. Soon you will notice a small door or opening, about the same size and shape as a mouse hole. Above the door is a sign saying, 'This way to the brain'.
>
> When you are ready, walk up to that small door and go through it. You find yourself looking at the base of your brain, and as you look at your brain, you notice that your hypothalamus gland is right there in front of you.
>
> As you stand there, take all the time you need to observe it really closely, using all of your senses to do so. Let yourself be curious about this part of the brain.
>
> Notice the colour. Is it bright and full of vigour or dull and lacking in vitality? Reach out and touch it. What does it feel like? Does it feel tense or calm? What is the texture like? Listen to the sounds it is producing. Does it sound tired? Breathe in and notice the smells. What does this tell you?
>
> Use all of your inner senses to discover the condition and needs of your hypothalamus. Take your time and be open to all the information which comes to you. Let yourself become aware of and learn about all the things that will be most useful for you. Allow yourself to become aware of the changes you can make to improve the healthy functioning of your hypothalamus.
>
> PAUSE

When you have all the information you need right now, thank your hypothalamus for being so co-operative. Turn round and go through the little door, back into the small room. In the small room you will notice on the wall a green button with the letter L for Large on it. When you are ready, press the green button and your body will get larger and larger until it returns to its normal size again.

*Source*
Adapted from James Schwartz (Schwartz, 2008, p. 63)

---

## *Bird Cage Release*

Can be done without formal hypnosis.

*Brief description*

This guided visualisation is set in a healing garden, using the metaphor of a bird trapped in a cage.

*Main aims*

- To resolve past events that may be affecting fertility.

- To release fears and emotions associated with miscarriage, termination and pregnancy.

*When would you use it?*

In *Stage 3: Resolve* for those who have previously miscarried or terminated a pregnancy and are finding it difficult to let go of the unhealthy emotions attached to it. In *Stage 5: Prepare* for clients to release fears about pregnancy, birth or parenthood.

*Contraindications*

- For those who may be pregnant
- Following transfer with IVF
- For clients who have a fear of birds.

*Script*

Lead the client into a healing garden and suggest that they find a comfortable place in the garden to rest.

As you rest in a comfortable place, feeling very calm and relaxed … you cast your eyes further around this wonderful lush garden … you notice in one area of the garden there is a beautiful bird cage … the most beautiful bird cage you have ever seen … perhaps it is made with intricate iron work or even simple wood … the cage intrigues you … and as you wander over to take a closer look … in the cage you notice a beautiful bird … it is calm and beautiful as it looks back at you … spend a little time getting to know the bird … looking at it closely … ask it how it feels in this cage … as you become aware of what this bird represents to you …

PAUSE

And you can begin to think about the possibility of opening the door of the cage … take your time … perhaps just opening the door slightly …

Spend a little time talking to the bird … tell the bird how you have been caring for it … and that sometimes you need to make space for something new … and now you need to let go … and release the bird …

Are you ready to set it free? … perhaps you don't yet feel ready … either is fine … just allow your unconscious mind to do whatever is safe and appropriate for you at this time …

PAUSE

If you want to speak to me and tell me what is happening that will be fine …

If the client is not yet ready to release the bird, you can suggest that they leave the door to the cage ajar so that they can revisit the bird in the following session/during *Self-Hypnosis*.

If they feel ready to release the bird:

Now that you are ready to release the bird … you can open the cage door fully … and let it go … making space for something new … allowing this to happen … watch with a sense of release as the bird flies off … perhaps staying close at first but then finding its own way … leaving a wonderful space in this fertile garden for something new … for something more appropriate for you at this time …

I will be quiet for a few moments while you ensure the space where your bird once sat is clear and prepared for something new …

PAUSE for a minute

It's time now to leave your healing garden … but this is a place you can visit anytime you wish … ensuring that there is space for something new and wonderful … leaving you free and open to new possibilities …

*How can it be adapted?*

This can be adapted by having a number of birds in the cage, each representing a negative thought or fear related to fertility/pregnancy and so on.

Clients who have either miscarried or terminated a pregnancy and feel they are in some way to blame, could release guilt by speaking to the bird and then letting it go.

*Source*
Contributed by Julie Cleasby, Clinical Hypnotherapist

# Cellular Memory Recall

*Brief description*

This technique uses IMRs to help the client consciously or unconsciously recall body memories of past conception and birth experiences. When the memories have been recalled the client is asked to take all the learnings from them so that they can once again conceive/have a baby. There is also an opportunity for the client to get insight into whether there are any conflicts arising from their desire to have a baby.

*Main aims*

- To restore trust and confidence in the body.
- To remind the client that they are 'capable' of having a baby and that conception/pregnancy is possible again.
- To resolve any parts conflicted with their desire to have a baby.

*When would you use it?*

This can be used in *Stage 3: Resolve* for those who have previously conceived or had a baby and can also be used to resolve any inner conflicts.

*Contraindications*

For those who are anxious that their mind and body may remember how to miscarry.

*Script*

> Install IMR finger signalling.
>
> And now I would like your inner mind to become fully aware … of its ability … to recall all of your experiences … all of those experiences that are retained at a deep cellular level … and it can be nice to know … that there is a memory deep within every cell in your body … that knows how to conceive … and how to develop a healthy pregnancy … and the birth of a beautiful baby … this may be a memory you have experienced …

or an unconscious memory passed down to you … from your ancestors … passed down in your DNA … and you may or may not consciously understand it or recall it fully …

And when you inner mind is fully aware of this cellular memory … there in your body … it can signal to me by lifting the Yes finger … take your time and trust in the process …

Wait for IMR.

And I would like your inner mind to take a few moments … to become fully aware of the positive and protective intent within this memory … become fully aware that cells, muscles and fibres can remember and know what to do … and when your inner mind has accessed these memories either at a cellular level … or an image level … or any other way that seems appropriate … it can signal to me by lifting the Yes finger …

Wait for IMR.

Now just spend a few moments accessing … in whatever way seems appropriate and right for you now … all of these memories in your own body … associated with being able to conceive … and conceiving successfully … I will go quiet to allow this process to happen …

PAUSE for a minute

When you have accessed those memories in the way that is appropriate for you … you can signal to me by lifting the Yes finger …

Wait for IMR.

That's good … now spend a few moments asking every area of your mind and body … if they are prepared to revisit and take on the learnings of these memories in order to help you conceive …

PAUSE

Now ask each area if there is any conflict with these memories … if there is any conflict about conceiving again? Take your time and trust in the process …

Spend time resolving any conflicts which arise.

Now that all areas are in agreement to conceive … fully taking on board the learnings of the past … to help conception in the future … just spend a few moments sending those valuable and wonderful memories … to every part of your mind … body … and spirit … in your own way … when every part is aware of these memories … you can let me know by lifting that Yes finger … and it's not important that you consciously know what those changes are until later …

Wait for IMR.

And you can be curious about which changes you will notice first …

*How can it be adapted?*

This can be used to recall cellular memory of any kind such as a past successful IVF.

*Source*
Contributed by Julie Cleasby BSc (Hons), Clinical Hypnotherapist, Dip. Clin. Hyp, NLP Prac.

---

## Healing White Light

Can be done without formal hypnosis.

*Brief description*

This visualisation uses white light to cleanse and clear the body and mind of anything that may be disturbing it. Once the light has cleared away any 'waste', it then brings health and wellbeing to the mind and body.

*Main aims*

- To cleanse and clear the mind-body.
- To restore balance and wellbeing.

The Fertile Body Method

*When would you use it?*

This approach could be used in *Stage 2: Balance* or *Stage 3: Resolve*. It may be useful for women who may have been trying to conceive for some time and have experienced numerous menstrual periods accompanied by disappointment and grief. Essentially it could be used to clear any mental, emotional or physical problems.

*Script*

> Make yourself comfortable … place your feet flat on the ground … and take a moment to just become aware of your breathing … the natural rhythm, the flow of life as you breathe in, and out … and as you continue to breathe … I want you to pay special attention to your body … just noticing how the air feels around your body … that cushion of air around your body … maybe it is getting a little warmer … pleasantly warm … as if being gently heated by a beautiful radiant sun … a beautiful golden sun above you … gently warming the air around your body … to a temperature that is just perfect for you.
>
> And as you allow the warmth of the sun … to help you relax a little deeper … so you can begin to be aware … of the light from the sun … streaming down … becoming a channel of white light … shining down on you … bathing your whole body in a cocoon of soft white light … continuing to warm your body … to a temperature that is just perfect for you … resting deeply … in the comforting soothing glow … aware of your breathing … sensing your whole body breathing…
>
> And now I'd like you to take in a slow deep breath … that's it … take a slow, deep breath … and as you breathe in… imagine that your skin is also taking a breath … breathing in the pure white light that surrounds you … that beautiful white light … and as you let your breath go … as you breathe out … I want you to imagine that your skin is also breathing out … and the light remains inside …
>
> … continue to breathe the light around you … continue to receive this purifying white light … that comes from deep within the sun … your whole body breathing … opening to receive this cleansing purifying white light … with each breath … the light flowing into your body … circulating throughout …
>
> PAUSE

Each breath is allowing that cleansing light to flow … more freely into your body … each breath drawing that white light into your body … cleansing each and every cell … purifying each and every cell … this beautiful light … drawn into every part of your body … clearing away disturbances, stagnation and blocks … leaving a feeling of wellbeing …

PAUSE

Feel your body being massaged … from the inside … as white light circulates … freely through your body … clearing and cleansing … deeply … easing out all the tension … all the tightness … creating a free flow of energy … as the old stagnation is washed away …

PAUSE

And the light can flow through your mind too … purifying white light … flowing through your current thoughts … through your past memories … flowing into all the stuck thoughts … into the mental blocks … into any frozen fears … softening them … loosening them … washing them away … leaving a feeling of calmness and clarity …

PAUSE

And all of the waste and debris … can be carried out of your body … down through your feet … and back into the earth … all of the tension and tightness can be washed away … down through your feet … and back to the earth … all of the old blocks can be washed away … into the earth … where it can become compost … where it can become fertiliser …

PAUSE

And when all the waste and debris has been cleared away … you can sense the light circulating more freely … free flowing radiant white light throughout … and as it moves through you and around you now … so it is bringing balance, harmony and wellbeing … so it is replenishing you …

Be aware of the white light flowing from the crown of your head … through your face and into your neck … restoring balance and harmony … now into your shoulders … your arms … into your hands … to the tips of your fingers … energising and restoring …

Down through your back and spine … renewing … invigorating … leaving a feeling of wellbeing, balance and vitality … and flowing through the front of your chest … down into your belly … bringing newness … and renewed hope … restoring every cell with a feeling of wellbeing …

Allow the light to flow down into your hips … bringing balance … brightness … through your legs and into your feet … energising … this vibrant white light … from the warming … healing sun …

PAUSE

Feel this life force pulsing through your body … creating the most wonderful feeling … of vitality and wellbeing now … taking a few moments … to allow yourself to receive this wisdom … from the sun… receive this pure source of vitality … on a deep unconscious level … feeling it inside of you and around you … enjoying its glow …

*Source*
Written by Sjanie Hugo

---

## Healing Green Light

Can be done without formal hypnosis.

*Brief description*

This visualisation uses a healing green light to induce deep relaxation. The green light emanates from within the earth and helps the client to connect more with nature and the natural creative life force.

*Main aims*

- To develop a connection with the earth and Mother Nature
- To increase confidence in their body

- To induce deep relaxation

- To enhance fertility.

*Script*

Make yourself comfortable … place your feet flat on the ground … and take a moment to just be aware of your breathing … the natural rhythm, flow of life as you breathe in, and out … and as you continue to breathe … I want you to pay special attention to your feet … just noticing how they feel … and allow your feet to sink a little more heavily into the ground beneath them … so that you can really start to feel the contact they make with the earth …

And imagine … that those feet are resting softly on the soil beneath them … and the soil can be cool or warm, creating just the right temperature … so that those feet can feel so comfortable, supported, resting there on this fertile earth … and as you breathe … just imagine that the soles of your feet are opening … to receive the most beautiful pulsating green light … that is coming from deep within the belly of the earth … the soles of your feet … opening to receive this nurturing, calming, pulsating green light … that is coming from deep within the earth … and is beginning to circulate up through those feet … and into your ankles … with every breath you take …

Each breath is allowing that life to flow … more freely into your body … each breath drawing that radiant green light up, up into your feet and ankles … and your legs now … and as it moves up it is relaxing and calming each and every cell … this beautiful nurturing green light … being drawn up through your ankles and legs … and you can breathe it up, right the way up into your hips … letting this pulsating green light fill the whole of your abdomen … deeply nourishing and nurturing you … bringing a wonderful sense of calm and relaxation …

Feel it circulating up through your feet … your legs and hips … through your belly … and then being draw up through the base of your spine … up each and every vertebra … just easing up … relaxing and calming … spreading all the way up to your neck … all the way up to the top of your head … then flowing down through your face … down through your arms, down the front of your body, all the way down … down into your hands … filling your hands, with this beautiful pulsating green light …

Each breath allows and invites this green light to circulate ... and flow freely through your whole body ... filling you with the most wonderful sense of calm and comfort ... feel the beautiful, nurturing embrace of this green light ... coming from deep within the earth ... and you can allow this light to really comfort you ... and nourish you ... in the most deep and satisfying way ...

Feeling this soft, beautiful green light flowing through your whole body ... feeling this pulsating strength, this life force that comes ... from deep with the earth ... this life force ... that gives birth to all life ... that sustains life ... that nourishes life ...

Feel this life force pulsing through your body ... creating the most wonderful feeling ... of comfort and strength now ... take a few moments ... to allow yourself to receive this wisdom ... this innate knowledge ... allow yourself on a deep, unconscious level ... to truly understand this creative force of life ... this natural force of life ... feeling it inside you and around you ... enjoying its beauty and strength ...

*Source*
Written by Sjanie Hugo

## *Creating A Fertile Body*

Can be done without formal hypnosis.

*Brief description*

This is a visualisation that encourages the client to engage more with their body and develop a better relationship with themself and their reproductive system. The client is also asked to talk to their body to find out what it needs in order to be in a healthy, fertile state. You can suggest that the client gives verbal answers to the questions or that they answer them silently.

*Main aims*

- To create a healthy relationship with their body

- To give their body more care and attention
- To become more conscious and aware of their body
- To develop a deeper understanding of their body
- To communicate with their body
- To prepare their body for conception
- To enhance fertility.

*When would you use it?*

Use this script for clients who seem to be very disconnected or detached from their body or for those who have a physical issue that may be affecting their fertility. It may be useful in *Stage 3: Resolve* to address any physical issues or in *Stage 4: Enhance*. This script can also get people to identify the changes they need to make in order to increase their chances of having a baby, and as such it may be used in *Stage 1: Outcome* to establish the goal for therapy.

*Script*

> I want you to become aware … that your body is made up of different parts … and each part of your body has its own unique function … its own speciality … and you can also become aware … that every part of your body is connected to its own set of memories … to its own history … for example … only your fingers can remember what it feels like to wash the dishes … your fingers can remember what it feels like to be in the warm soapy water … and each finger has its own unique individual memory … of each of those experiences …
>
> Every part of your body holds within it … a complete set of memories … sensations, experiences and knowledge … and if you pay attention … you will also begin to notice that you have a different relationship with these different parts of your body … for example, the way you feel about your feet … the way you think of your feet … is very different to the way you feel about your ears … what you think about your ears …
>
> With each and every part of your body … you have a unique relationship … and some parts of your body you know really well … and other parts not so well … Some parts of your body you give a lot of attention to …

## The Fertile Body Method

and others you pay very, very little attention ... but right now, at this time of your life ... your attention is being called down to the organs of your reproductive system ... to that inner part ... down there below your belly ... your ovaries ... your womb ... and each part has its own memories and experiences ... and you may have given them some attention many, many times before ... or perhaps not at all. You may have noticed how hard they've been working for you ... each and every month ... or perhaps barely noticed them ...

*What I want you to do now... is to become aware of your reproductive system... and pay special attention to your womb ...

How do you perceive this part of your body ... is it big or small ... long or wide ... dark or light ... spacious or cramped ... is it hard or soft ... friendly or unfriendly?

PAUSE

When you think about your womb ... how do you feel?

PAUSE

Notice the nature of your relationship to your womb ... perhaps an image comes to mind that best describes the nature of your relationship to this part of your body?

PAUSE

And now ask that part of your body what it needs from you.

Some people find that they need to give their womb more nurturing ... more love ... some people find they need to talk to it ... pay it more attention ... and like all relationships ... you will find that the more attention you give this part of your body ... the better the relationship becomes ... like all relationships ... the more attention you give it ... the better it becomes ... and so you can begin ... to find ways to pay attention to this part of your body ... more and more ... every day ...

By asking what it needs ... by giving it what it needs ... by noticing it more ... thinking about it more ... feeling it more ... loving it more ... perhaps massaging it ... talking to it ... imagining it ... and the more attention you give it ... the better it feels ... the more it responds ... the better your relationship becomes ... and the more ready and available it becomes … and what you are doing … is creating a nurturing, loving safe environment conducive to life … you are creating a healthy fertile state …

(To continue working with another part of the reproductive system, such as the ovaries, return to* and adapt the script accordingly.)

*How can it be adapted?*

This can be adapted for any organ or system in the body. The script above refers to the female reproductive system but it can, of course, be adapted for men. It can be used to help increase the effectiveness of drugs by communicating with the relevant body parts to find out what changes would support the medication.

*Source*
Written by Sjanie Hugo

---

## Connect With Your Inner Body

Can be done without formal hypnosis.

*Brief description*

This is a deeply relaxing visualisation that connects the client with their inner body and the life force within them. The client is directed to focus on their reproductive system to restore balance and rhythm.

*Main aims*

- To create hormonal balance
- To regulate the rhythms of the body
- To regulate the menstrual cycle
- To increase reproductive health and wellbeing

## The Fertile Body Method

- To encourage deep relaxation
- To deepen body awareness.

*When would you use it?*

Useful for anyone with hormonal problems, specifically those with irregular menstrual cycles. Since it produces a deep state of relaxation and helps to regulate the body's equilibrium, it may be used in *Stage 2: Balance* or in *Stage 4: Enhance*. For those with menstrual health problems it may help to resolve these issues in *Stage 3: Resolve*.

*Script*

> Allow your mind to make contact with your body ... at first making contact with the weight and stillness of your physical form ... feeling the density and gravity of your solid quiet body ... let the peace and tranquility deepen ... as you pay more attention to your body ...
>
> Now allow your mind ... to make contact with the inside of your body ... let yourself become aware of the movement that's happening inside ... feel and sense the fluid and flowing nature of your inner body ... feel more deeply inside your body ... so that you can feel the force of life ... that brings movement to every cell ... enjoy the deep breath ... that brings change and motion ... perhaps you can even be aware ... of the sound of your heart beating inside your chest ...
>
> Begin now ... to get a sense of what your body looks like ... from the inside ... focus your attention on your abdominal area ... become more aware of your uterus ... Fallopian tubes and ovaries ... start to feel the rhythm that governs these organs ... let your awareness expand ... to include your brain and hypothalamus ... pituitary gland ... cervix ... and vagina ... notice how these different parts are all in constant communication with each other ... sending messengers through the system ... giving each part instructions about what it needs to do when ... and everything can happen in perfect timing ... because the whole of this system knows how to be in perfect balance and harmony ... It also listens to the cycles of nature ... all around you ... and knows how to follow the lead of the moon ... and as you consider these messengers ... these hormones ... balanced and working in perfect harmony ... your level of relaxation can deepen ...

As you allow your unconscious mind … to trace the whole of your reproductive system now … you can start to feel more and more deeply relaxed … there is nothing you need to do … your unconscious mind knows how to regulate the systems of your body … and your unconscious mind knows how to create a natural synchronicity and rhythm in your reproductive system … And as you continue to enjoy the rhythm of my words … so your body is enjoying its own rhythm … enjoying a regular monthly rhythm …

*How can it be adapted?*

This can be adapted for any system of the body and can be used for men or women.

*Source*
Written by Sjanie Hugo

## Tune Into Your Body Clock

Can be done without formal hypnosis.

*Brief description*

This visualisation guides the client into a sanctuary where their body clock is housed. They are invited to make any repairs or adjustments needed to restore their body clock and the natural rhythm of their reproductive system.

*Main aims*

- To restore regularity and rhythm to the body
- To create menstrual health
- To create hormonal balance.

The Fertile Body Method

*When would you use it?*

This script would be beneficial for anyone who is experiencing disruptions to their bodily rhythms, which could include those with sleep problems, digestive issues or menstrual health problems. It can be used in *Stage 2: Balance* to restore rhythm or in *Stage 3: Resolve* to resolve problems that are connected to a disruption of body rhythms.

*Script*

> Imagine that you are walking down a bright radiant tunnel … which leads towards the sanctuary where your body clock is housed … when you come to the end of the tunnel … you arrive at this beautiful sanctuary … the rhythm of life is inescapable … everything in this place is pulsing with this life … perhaps you can even hear this rhythm as a soulful ticking … let yourself be drawn towards the place where your body clock is kept … let the pulsing … ticking rhythm of life … draw you towards the clock …
>
> As you get closer … pay attention to the way your body ticks … the sound of your own internal clock … this is your master clock … it governs all the other smaller clocks … that are housed in the different organs and tissues of your body … the sunlight that streams in through that tunnel … really helps to keep this master clock in sync with the external world …
>
> This master clock … governs the smaller clocks in your reproductive system … notice now how this master clock does that … notice how it can instruct the other clocks … and how it can ensure that your menstrual cycle is regular …
>
> While in this sanctuary … you can do some essential maintenance work … that can restore this clock … and get it back into good condition … do whatever you need to do now … to ensure that your reproductive clock is fully synchronised with your master clock … ensure that the clocks are ticking in perfect rhythm … when you can see, hear or feel that inner harmony and rhythm … and feel that your body clocks are working well … let me know …

*Source*
Written by Sjanie Hugo

## *Fertility Garden*

Can be done without formal hypnosis.

*Brief description*

This visualisation is a metaphorical approach that guides the client into their *Fertility Garden* and suggests that they clear the weeds that are growing there. Once they have removed the weeds, they then plant new seeds and spend some time resting and rejuvenating in their garden.

*Main aims*

- To 'de-weed' and clear any beliefs, feelings or experiences which may be affecting fertility.
- To 'plant' new beliefs, feelings and behaviours which will enhance fertility.

*When would you use it?*

In *Stage 3: Resolve* to release conscious or unconscious resistance to having a baby and in *Stage 4: Enhance*.

*Script*

- Imagine walking along a path until you reach a wall in which there is a door, in your hand you find a key that unlocks the door.
- Walk through the door into a beautiful garden; this is your fertility garden.
- Notice what it looks like, what it sounds like, the aromas, what is growing there and so on.
- Look around the garden and as you do you notice a patch of weeds; go over to the place where the weeds are growing.
- In your garden you find weedkiller, tools for digging, fresh earth, fertiliser and new seeds.
- Dig up, pull up or kill the weeds and prepare the soil for new seeds.
- You can let me know when this is done.

- PAUSE
- Now you can plant your new seeds and water them.
- Once this is done you can find somewhere to rest and relax in the garden.
- You can relax deeply knowing that you have done all the work you need to do and those seeds have now been planted in your fertility garden.
- All you now need to do is continue to nurture those seeds, and in time they will grow.
- As you rest in the garden, you can start to imagine all the ways in which you can nurture yourself.
- Each time you nurture yourself, each time you take care of yourself, so you are watering the seeds and encouraging new life to grow and prosper.
- Take some time to rest and relax in the garden as you daydream about the ways in which you will nourish yourself and these seeds.
- After some ego strengthening suggestions, guide them back to the door.
- As you leave the garden you lock the door behind you, knowing that you can return here whenever you choose.
- Guide them back along the path to re-orientate them.
- Awaken.

*Source*
Adapted from the work of Milton H. Erickson, M.D.

---

## *IVF Preparation*

Can be done without formal hypnosis.

*Brief description*

This visualisation combines aspects of the *Primal Image* to help clients imagine their ovaries and uterus responding well to the IVF treatment. Suggestions are given for them to imagine their ovaries producing good-quality eggs and for their womb to thicken and prepare to receive the fertilised embryos.

*Main aims*

- To prepare the client for IVF
- To increase the effectiveness of the medication
- To decrease negative side effects from IVF medication
- To build confidence.

*When would you use it?*

Use this in *Stage 4: Prepare* to prepare the client for IVF treatment. It can also be used as a visualisation during stimulation and before embryo transfer.

*Script*

> Your body can rest deeply now … so that you can communicate with your unconscious mind … to create some positive changes to the way you think and feel … to the way your body responds … just letting your body rest deeply for this time now … as you allow yourself to become aware of your ovaries … just noticing what image comes to mind as you connect with, and become aware of your ovaries … starting to see the shape, colours, textures … just noticing how your ovaries appear to you right now … letting that become clear in your mind as if it were an image on your inner screen which you can see clearly …
>
> And then recognising you have all the tools you need … you have all the colours in the rainbow available to you … the brushes and the tools, just as if you are an artist … and you can begin to make whatever changes you need to make … so that those ovaries look healthy, fertile and full of life … perhaps changing the colour or texture, the size or the detail … doing whatever you need to do … so that you can see those ovaries youthful and full of life … with follicles containing good-quality eggs, each egg filled with the potential for life …
>
> So you can see those ovaries healthy and vital … and know that each time you take your medication … it's like a golden light being absorbed by your body … and that medication, that beautiful golden light … can go to the parts of your body that need it most … and perhaps you can see that golden light flowing towards those ovaries … stimulating them,

encouraging them … filling and penetrating those ovaries with golden light so that they produce good-quality eggs … just the right number of good-quality healthy eggs … and any extra, surplus golden light can easily be let go… released from your body … and you need not experience any negative side effects … as any surplus can be let go and carried away … as those ovaries receive that golden light of encouragement … just as much as they need to produce good-quality eggs …

And imagine those ovaries are fertile, alive, producing good-quality eggs … and allow that image to sink back deep into your unconscious mind … and then become aware of your womb … connecting with your womb, your uterus, allowing an image to come to mind as you think about your womb … so that you can get a clear sense of your womb in your mind's eye … just as it appears right now, noticing its size … shape … noticing any colours … become aware of the textures … noticing the temperature … the atmosphere that's inside … as you prepare your womb to receive those healthy fertilised embryos …

You can use the tools you have, the colours, the brushes the textures you need … first make that womb really safe … make it a safe place, a safe womb that can easily and effortlessly hold and protect your baby … making that womb totally safe … using colour, using texture doing it in whatever way is right for you … and as you prepare this womb to receive these fertilised embryos … you can ensure that this womb is nurturing and nourishing … making any changes you need to now make sure that this womb is nurturing and nourishing … that your baby will receive all the nutrients it needs … all the oxygen, the fresh blood supply that will encourage that fertilised embryo to implant … to grow to thrive … so that you can see that womb now … safe and nurturing and nourishing too …

And finally do whatever you need to do … to make that womb welcoming and inviting … so when that baby arrives in this place … this place that will be their home for nine months … they will feel welcome and wanted … making this womb welcoming and inviting and infuse it with love … that unconditional love that a mother can have for a baby … before they've even been conceived … infuse it with that love, that warmth … so your womb is safe and nurturing … so that it's welcoming and loving too …

Make a comfortable and warming place … so that when you receive those fertilised embryos they can implant into the thick, lush lining of your womb … and you can see that embryo dividing rapidly … cells dividing and multiplying … that embryo growing bigger and bigger … all the while your body nourishing and nurturing that growing life … that baby is beginning to develop and grow … in that safe, nurturing, warm, comfortable home …

Your womb full of life … full of growth, full of possibility … and then let that sink back deeply into your unconscious mind … and allow yourself to rest in that quiet place … and anything you need right now … any help that you need, any healing that you need … it can come to you in this place … taking whatever form is appropriate …

Just allow yourself now to be open to receive whatever you need … seeing it, feeling it, sensing it … as your mind, your heart and your body receive whatever it is they need right now … to bring you peace, to bring you stillness, to bring you strength … and you can rest, knowing that you have done everything you can … you can rest, at peace … and you can be open, you can be open to the possibilities that lie ahead … knowing that you deserve good things … knowing that you can be a mother … and that you can be a good mother … that you can love and care for and nurture a growing child … and that you deserve to be happy and content and fulfilled … and sooner or later you can be a mother … and you can enjoy that contentment … and as you allow that all to sink deep inside … feeling a wonderful sense of calmness right the way through …

*Source*
Written by Sjanie Hugo

## Embryo Transfer

Can be done without formal hypnosis.

*Brief description*

This visualisation guides the client into their womb to prepare it for the arrival of their embryos. They are asked to imagine the embryo/s arriving and implanting in the womb. In cases where the client has more than one embryo put back the script should be adjusted accordingly.

The Fertile Body Method

Use a deep relaxation script such as *Breathing Colour* before this *Embryo Transfer* visualisation to help the client achieve a good state of relaxation.

*Main aims*

- To support women during IVF embryo transfer
- To prepare the womb for implantation
- To create deep relaxation
- To increase blood flow to the uterus.

*When would you use it?*

Use this with women undergoing IVF treatment in the days leading up to embryo transfer and/or during embryo transfer.

*Script*

> And as you drift deeper and deeper, more relaxed … you can become aware of your womb … just allow yourself to drift even deeper now, so that you can drift down, down inside your womb … so that you can drift deep into the heart of your womb … and as you do … you can feel more calm … and more relaxed …
>
> Relaxing deeply now … allowing yourself to just get a sense of what it's like to be in this amazing place … this spectacular womb that has the capacity to hold life … that has the capacity to nurture growing life … this wonderfully comfortable, safe and nurturing place deep inside you … where you can be aware of the sound of your own heart beating … very softly, very rhythmically … there in the background … providing a rhythm of comfort and reassurance …
>
> And as you let yourself rest here in the heart of your womb … you can take a moment to prepare this place for the arrival of your baby … to prepare this place so that is warm and welcoming … so that your womb looks and feels really comfortable and inviting … so that it feels really cosy and nurturing …
>
> You're preparing your womb room now to receive your fertilised embryo … and from deep inside this place you can prepare to meet your

## Techniques, Scripts and Tools

embryo… to welcome your baby to its new home … feeling yourself becoming more ready and prepared … welcoming your embryo … welcoming your baby to its new home …

PAUSE

You can really get a sense of that embryo arriving into this womb … and know that it's been longing to come here … to this safe and inviting place … this is where it belongs … notice how it can float … safely inside that womb … until it's time to comfortably embed into the thick, lush lining … and you can get a sense of that embryo comfortably embedding in your womb … tucking up safely … as millions of tiny capillaries connect with your womb … and the lining of your uterus is thick and lush and nutritious … creating a wonderfully safe and nurturing environment …

And you can become aware of the connections that will begin to develop … that intricate network of blood vessels … growing more and more with each passing moment … and with each moment your baby is continuing to create connections with you through your blood … your fluid … and that growing umbilical cord … and in each passing moment … every day… these connections are growing stronger and stronger …

That wonderful intelligence that is deep within you … knows how to nurture this growing baby… and you can trust your body more and more … trusting that your body knows how to do this …

PAUSE

Just think now about the child you want to give birth to … and allow that vision … of that beautiful, healthy baby … to encourage and nurture this life that is growing within you … in each passing moment as you think about that baby you want to give birth to … hold that vision clear and strong in your mind and let it be a guiding light, that encourages and nurtures your baby through each passing moment … through each day … and each stage of pregnancy … right the way through to the day of its birth …

PAUSE

And whenever you think of your womb now … you can be aware of it as a wonderful place … a fertile, nourishing and creative place … vibrant, full of life … and you can see your baby growing … comfortable and safe … being nurtured and nourished … receiving everything it needs to grow and thrive ... all the while you can feel peaceful and at ease ... feeling a sense of ever deepening calm and trust ... knowing that everything will work out exactly how it needs to ... feeling an ever-deepening trust in the process of life ... in the wonderful timing of all things ... and allow this calmness to be with you in the days and weeks ahead ... to comfort you ... helping you to feel relaxed and at ease ... (REPEAT THIS PARAGRAPH.)

*Source*
Written by Sjanie Hugo

---

## *Implantation*

Can be done without formal hypnosis.

*Brief description*

This visualisation guides the client to imagine a fertilised embryo implanting into the thick lining of the womb.

*Main aims*

- To support and enhance implantation
- To create increased body awareness
- To build a bond/connection between the mother and the embryo
- To build the client's trust and confidence in their body.

*When would you use it?*

During *Stage 4: Enhance* this visualisation can be used to enhance natural or assisted conception. During IVF treatment it can be used pre- and post-transfer as an alternative to the *Embryo Transfer* script. It's also useful for women who are using donated embryos to help them connect and bond with the embryos.

## Script

As you become aware of your womb now … just allow yourself to go a little deeper … drift a little deeper now … drift deep inside … to meet your embryo … and welcome your baby to its new home …

PAUSE

And as you begin to imagine being deep inside your womb … you can start to get a sense of that fertilised embryo … comfortably embedded in your womb … perhaps imagining what it looks like as it implants into the folds of your soft uterus wall … in that warmth and comfort … where all the conditions are perfect for life to grow and flourish …

PAUSE

And in every moment that embryo is growing and developing … the outer layers, penetrating your uterus … imbedding into the soft comfortable lining … like roots sinking deep into the fertile soil … where they can receive the nourishment that they need … the soft thick lining of your womb…is lush and nutritious … providing your growing baby with all of the nutrients and oxygen it needs …

And as the placenta develops … and that intricate network of blood vessels … grows more and more with each passing moment … so your baby is continuing to create connections with you … through your blood … through your fluids and through the growing umbilical cord … each day these connections are growing stronger and stronger …

And your body instinctively knows how to respond … to your baby's needs … giving your baby exactly what is needed … feeding and nourishing your growing baby … encouraging the cells to continue to divide … supporting your baby in every way … as your body supports those cells to grow … in a healthy and vital way …

PAUSE

You can begin to think now … about the child you want to give birth to … and allow that vision … to encourage and nurture your baby … through each passing moment …

PAUSE

And you can use your thoughts in a powerful way … use your thoughts in a powerful way to tell your baby, 'I want you and I love you' … just creating that gentle and intimate bond … strengthening the connection that is already there … that very deep and loving connection … and tell your baby, 'I'm creating a loving environment for you now and for always' …

And in every moment, with each and every thought, feeling and experience … you are inviting these connections to grow stronger and stronger … together you're growing more and more … together you're creating … together you're growing stronger and stronger … with each passing day … deepening that bond … strengthening that connection … nourishing that life … in a very healthy and vital way …

*Source*
Inspired by Maggie Chapman
Written by Sjanie Hugo

---

## **The Mirror of Forgiveness**

Can be done without formal hypnosis.

*Brief description*

This visualisation guides the client to work with a mirror of forgiveness which has the capacity to release their guilt and bring forgiveness and peace.

*Main aims*

- To release guilt
- To create forgiveness
- To resolve the negative effects of past events.

Techniques, Scripts and Tools

*When would you use it?*

In *Stage 3: Resolve* to address any past experiences associated with guilt and self-blame, for example termination of pregnancy.

*Script*

Lead the client into a healing garden and suggest that they find a comfortable place in the garden to rest.

- As you rest in the garden you notice a twinkling light in between the flowers.
- Feel yourself becoming more curious until eventually you wander towards the sparkling glimmer.
- As you get closer you see that it is a magical mirror.
- Sit down in front of the mirror.
- And notice the beautiful frame of this magical mirror.
- And as you do you will see your reflection looking back at you.
- Your reflection is smiling kindly at you.
- Your reflection begins to speak, telling you that this is the 'Mirror Of Forgiveness' and anything that is revealed to this mirror can be forgiven.
- Take some time, now, to talk to the mirror, telling her all about your experience.
- Explain to the mirror, why you did what you did.
- PAUSE
- Ask for forgiveness.
- And as you do, your beautiful reflection looks back at you.
- Her eyes are filled with compassion, she understands completely.
- Then she tells you that all has been forgiven.
- Feel the weight lifting as you receive that forgiveness.

Suggest that the client spends some time resting and relaxing in their garden, allowing this healing to sink in deeply.

*Source*
Written by Sjanie Hugo
Inspired by a client. See the case study: *indirectly resolving issues* (Page 90).

The Fertile Body Method

## *The Big Race*

*Brief description*

This visualisation asks men to imagine their sperm in a race to reach the egg which only one sperm will penetrate and fertilise.

*Main aims*

- To increase sperm mobility and morphology
- To build testosterone
- To increase potency
- To build confidence.

*When would you use it?*

This could be used in *Stage 4: Enhance* and is particularly useful for men with sperm problems.

*Script*

> I would like you to imagine the start of a race … the start of a very important race … and it doesn't matter what kind of race it is … it could be the start of a Formula 1 car race … the drivers waiting in their cars, the roar of the powerful engines as they prepare for the starter's flag … or it could even be the beginning of the 100 metre sprint … the athletes in their starting blocks … the visible strength and power in their muscles, as they wait for the sound of the pistol … and when you've pictured the start of a race … what I want you to do, is really look at it … try and imagine what it might feel like to be there … to see these healthy, confident athletes … or the fearless and determined drivers … every single one of them ready for their race … a race that each one of them is prepared for … a race that each one of them knows that they can win … I want you to try and feel their confidence … their strength … as it radiates from each and every one of them … as they wait at the starting line … wait for the start of the race.

And I now want you to take that feeling … that feeling of strength and power … and imagine that it is your sperm at the start of their own race … see your sperm as the incredible athletes they are … at the start of their own race … see how strong they are … how confident … how pumped up and ready to go … feel their determination and strength, as it radiates from them … like lean, aerodynamic racing vehicles … fantastic athletes … ready to propel themselves along their course …

And I'd like you to just focus on their determination … feel their power … each and every one of them ready for the race … a race that each one of them is trained for … built for … prepared for … a race that each one of them believes they can win … and when you are ready … I want you to start the race … and it doesn't matter how you do it … just start the race … start the race and let them go … a perfect start …

Now … imagine them racing through the slippery cervix, their powerful tails propelling them faster and faster at incredible speed … each one getting stronger and stronger … more and more powerful … as they ride on the lubricated surface, fighting for position and not one of them giving any ground … every single one of them wanting to win … determined to win … I want you to feel their strength … see their potential … and know that it is your strength … your determination … that is pushing them forward.

Then watch as they reach the uterus … a group of incredible athletes, still pushing faster and faster forward, knowing instinctively which direction they need to go in … choosing instinctively which tube they need to pick … and as they race forward they are becoming more and more focused … as if each one of them knows that the finish line is in sight … each one focused on victory … each one pushing harder to be the winner … see how fast they are going … see how strong and powerful they are … how determined … and confident.

The egg is now in sight … and every single one of your sperm is increasing its speed … its desire … and its power is multiplied

TEN TIMES … TWENTY TIMES … as each one pushes for position … battling to be the strongest sperm that penetrates the egg … then they reach it … reach the egg … and one sperm pushes harder … thrusting itself forward, deep into the egg … penetrating it … winning the race … the victor … the strongest athlete … amongst the strongest collection of athletes you have ever seen … the best of best…

and now you can imagine the victorious sperm pushing itself further into the egg ... with more desire than ever ... so alive with energy and strength ... see your sperm reaching the centre of the egg ... fusing with the egg ... bursting into life ... becoming one ... a magical mass of new life ... of energy ... of strength ... as your DNA combines with her DNA ... forming something new ... something totally unique...

And perhaps you can begin to imagine ... how the combination of her perfect egg and your winning sperm ... will grow ... grow into your beautiful ... healthy ... child ...

*How can it be adapted?*

It can be adapted for women to imagine her partner's sperm. This is especially useful for a woman whose partner has had sperm problems.

*Source*
Written by Sjanie Hugo

## **Conception**

*Brief description*

This visualisation guides the client to imagine the moment of conception and the biological process of embryo development.

*Main aims*

- To increase understanding of the biological process of conception and the stages of development.

- To enhance fertility and build confidence.

*When would you use it?*

This could be used in *Stage 4: Enhance* to enhance natural conception or it could be adapted and used to enhance medical treatments such as IUI, IVF and Donation.

*Contraindications*

For those who have previously miscarried after the 12 weeks scan, thinking about the baby's heartbeat may be contraindicated.

*Script*

> I wonder if you have ever imagined … what it would be like … to be able to see the moment in which your baby is conceived … to be able to zoom in on that special egg … so that you can see the victorious sperm … penetrating the outer layer … and reaching the centre … bursting into life … fusing together … becoming one … that moment of union … when new life begins … a magical mass of new life … of energy … containing all the necessary information and potential to grow into a baby … into a totally unique human being …
>
> And I wonder if you have ever imagined … what it would be like … to be able to watch that new life grow … as the cells divide … and multiply … as that zygote travels down your Fallopian tube … caressed and encourage by the tiny hair-like cilia in the tube … cells dividing and multiplying as it moves … down the Fallopian tube … and then arriving … in your womb …
>
> And if you could see this new life… this ball of cells … with an outer shell … arriving in your womb … you would be able to see how the outer shell develops into the placenta … and the inner cells develop into the embryo … and within a week or so … this blastocyst attaches itself to the lining of your womb … finding just the right place … to settle in comfortably …
>
> And you would see the lining thick and lush … and ready to support this new life … ready to support this growing life … ready to give nourishment through your bloodstream …

And I'm not sure if you know … that once the embryo has formed … and the cells have multiplied further … the cells begin to take on specific functions … some become blood cells … others become kidney cells, nerve cells, brain cells and so on … growing rapidly … as every cell needed to create a human being develops …

And if you were watching now … you would start to see … your baby's main features beginning to take form … new, yet familiar … your baby's beautiful features forming …

And after eight weeks … everything is ready to just grow and develop … grow and develop … and by 12 weeks … your baby will be filling your womb … nestled in safely … growing and developing …

And perhaps you can imagine … that special moment … when you hear your baby's heart beat for the first time … when the life that has been growing inside … can be heard …

*Source*
Written by Sjanie Hugo

## SELF-HELP TOOLS

This section describes a range of self-help tools that can be taught to the client. These tools vary from practical tasks to various applications of self-hypnosis. the self-help tools form the basics of the between session 'homework'. Self-help tools are a valuable part of the *Fertile Body Method* because they can:

- Reinforce the work done during the session

- Help the client to develop new skills

- Develop the clients self-awareness

- Generate information for both the client and practitioner

- Assist the client's learning by means of using the self-help tools

- Create physiological change, e.G. Boost the immune system, balance the hormones, induce relaxation

- Motivate the client to take steps or actions towards their goal

- Prepare for an upcoming event

- Maintain change.


Below is a selection of tasks and self-help tools that I have found to be valuable in helping to create change. Each tool includes a description, step-by-step guide on how to do it and examples of when it can be used. It is best to teach the self-help tool to your client in the session and then give them a handout (available on the CD) to remind them about what they have learnt and how to use it.

- Self-Hypnosis .................................................................................281
- Mini-Break Anchor .......................................................................282
- Mindfulness ...................................................................................282
- Orange Dots ..................................................................................283
- Affirmations ..................................................................................283
- Grief Ceremony / Ceremony To Say Goodbye .........................284
- Meditation .....................................................................................285
- Mental Rehearsal ..........................................................................286
- Creative Tasks ...............................................................................287
- Gratitudes ......................................................................................288

- Menstrual Diary ...................................................................................288
- 7:11 Breathing .......................................................................................289
- Quick Body Scan ..................................................................................289
- Emotional Bank Account ....................................................................290
- Nurturing ...............................................................................................290
- Cognitive Restructuring .....................................................................291
- Self-Talk SUDS .....................................................................................292
- Polarity Exercise ..................................................................................293

## Self-Hypnosis

*Self-Hypnosis* should be taught while the patient is in a trance state. There are many different ways to teach *Self-Hypnosis* and the therapist should select the method that works best for the client. Suggestions to easily learn to enter this state on their own can be given before awakening the client.

*An example of how to do Self-Hypnosis*

- Close your eyes
- Focus on your breathing
- Silently and mentally count down from ten to one
- Count on every second out-breath
- As you exhale and count each number, let your body become more relaxed
- As you count ten, focus on your head and face, and let them relax
- As you count nine, focus on your neck and shoulders, and let them relax
- As you count eight, focus on your arms and hands and let them relax
- As you count seven, focus on your upper back and let it relax
- As you count six, focus on your chest and let it relax
- As you count five, focus on your belly and lower back, and let them relax
- As you count four, focus on your pelvis and hips, and let them relax
- As you count three, focus on your thighs and knees, and let them relax
- As you count two, focus on your calves and ankles, and let them relax
- As you count one, focus on your feet and toes, and let them relax
- When in this relaxed state the client can rest and enjoy the benefits of this relaxation, do a positive visualisation or repeat an affirmation.

This state can also be used to practise any other techniques the therapist may have taught the client in a session.

*The long-term benefits of Self-Hypnosis*

According to the Mind Body Institute in California, *Eliciting the relaxation response 20 minutes per day for 2–6 weeks will increase levels of calmness and relaxation in everyday life, as well as increase health.* (The Mind Body Institute, http://www.mindbodyinfertility.com)

## Mini-Break Anchor

The *Mini-Break Anchor* is a rapid way to take the edge off anxiety and to clear the mind and restore a sense of control. Mini-Breaks can be done to prevent emotional distress. The *Mini-Break* can be anchored to the deep relaxation achieved using *10 to 1 Self-Hypnosis*.

*How to take a Mini-Break*

- Place your hands on your abdomen, just on top of your belly button. This will remind you to breathe deeply and relax your stomach muscles.
- Breathe in slowly and deeply.
- Pause after the in-breath.
- As you exhale, silently count from ten to zero.
- Do this for a few breaths or until you feel the tension leaving.

(Domar, 2002, p. 61)

---

## Mindfulness

*Mindfulness* is a practice that comes from the Buddhist tradition. It is a state of observation and awareness that allows you to appreciate the here and now. *Mindfulness* connects you with the present moment, which is free from suffering. It reconnects you with simple pleasures. For some it may work as a reminder that the world is more than just 'trying to have a baby' and can increase feelings of relaxation.

*How to engage in mindful activity*

- Give all of your attention to whatever it is you are doing: it could be something as simple as walking or washing the dishes.
- Do it slowly.
- Fully experience the physical sensations.
- Focus on allowing each of your senses to take in the surroundings.
- Become aware of all the details via your senses.
- When thoughts intrude on your awareness, gently return your focus on the sensations, smells, sounds and sights.
- Remain in a state of non-judgement.
- Simply allow yourself to receive the moment.

## Orange Dots

The *Orange Dot* is literally an orange dot sticker that can be stuck somewhere where it can be seen on a regular basis throughout the day. The dot acts as a cue/trigger to remind you to carry out a particular task. Tasks can include anything from repeating an affirmation or visualisation to taking a deep, relaxing breath.

*How to use the Orange Dots as a therapeutic tool*

Affirmations are a very effective way of reinforcing healthy beliefs and creating inner change. The orange dot cue can provide a self-help tool that will trigger a reminder to repeat this affirmation on a regular basis.

During the hypnotic session, the therapist can establish the trigger by making the following suggestion:

> And whenever you see that orange dot that you have now stuck onto your purse, you will repeat your belief, 'I trust my body's natural capacity to create life' silently and mentally to yourself. And each time you do this, so your trust is growing allowing your body to respond as soon as it is ready …

---

## Affirmations

An affirmation is:

- A positively phrased statement to yourself
- Phrased in the present tense
- Simple and short
- A statement that starts with the word 'I/My/ …'

Examples:

> *I am becoming more and more confident in myself.*
> *I am choosing healthy food that makes me feel good.*
> *I love and appreciate my body.*

The practice of doing affirmations allows you to begin replacing some of your stale, worn-out or negative mind chatter with more positive ideas and concepts. It is a powerful technique, one that can in a short time completely transform your attitudes and expectations about life, and thereby totally change what you experience.

Traditionally, an affirmation is a positive statement to oneself. However, simply saying the statement to oneself while feeling quite the opposite of what is being said produces an incongruent state that sometimes can be less than helpful. In order for an affirmation to be useful, it needs to be embodied as if it were happening now. In this way you are actually creating (although temporarily) a congruent and evocative experience of the change that you want. By repeatedly accessing the words, emotions and physical state you begin to learn this way of being.

Seeking to verify the truth of this statement in our day-to-day life can also help this statement become a deep-seated belief.

*How to use an Affirmation*

- Take some time to settle down and relax.
- Allow your eyes to close.
- Say the affirmation to yourself out loud and continue to repeat it several more times.
- As you continue to say the affirmation, start to imagine that it is already true.
- Imagine it as if it were happening now.
- Imagine the feelings and emotions that you will be experiencing.
- Imagine how your body will be feeling and moving.
- Where possible, physically perfom the movement or adopt the posture.
- Let yourself fully embody this statement in every way.

---

## *Grief Ceremony / Ceremony To Say Goodbye*

A *Grief Ceremony* can help you process and mourn the loss of your unborn child. Irrespective of whether you have lost a child due to miscarriage, abortion, still-birth or infertility, creating a ritual to say goodbye allows you to acknowledge the loss and emotionally release your unborn child (Payne and Richardson, 2002). The most powerful ceremonies will always be the ones which you create because they will be more meaningful to you. You could do the ceremony alone or with you partner or a close friend.

*How to hold a Grief Ceremony*

Follow these guidelines and suggestions for creating a simple yet meaningful ritual for saying goodbye.

- Gather any objects which remind you of your unborn baby. These can be items such as scans, cards from friends, gifts, pregnancy tests or you may choose a symbolic object such as a flower, doll or balloon.
- Write a letter to your unborn child. In the letter you may write about what their life meant to you, how you feel about the loss, why you are doing this ceremony and saying goodbye. Or you may prefer to find a poem or a story which you would like to read at the ceremony.
- Find a special place to do your ceremony. You may choose to do it in your garden, at home, near a river, or by the sea.
- Prepare the space. You could decorate it, light candles, place flowers, put on some music and create a comfortable place to sit.
- Take some time to sit in silence, to relax and focus your intention.
- When you are ready read the letter, poem or story out loud. Say any words which are meaningful for you.
- Allow as much time as you need to say goodbye.
- Find a symbolic ritual to say goodbye. You may want to release a balloon, bury the items you have brought or burn the letter.
- Find a symbolic ritual to give thanks. You may like to plant a flower or sprinkle some seeds. This is an opportunity for you to give thanks for whatever you can.
- Close the ceremony.

## Meditation

*Meditation* is a mental discipline during which you attempt to get beyond the conditioned 'thinking' mind into a deeper state of relaxation or awareness. Meditation often involves turning attention to a single point of reference. There are many different meditation techniques.

*How to practise a simple breathing meditation*

- Choose a quiet place and sit in a comfortable position. You can sit in a chair or in the traditional cross-legged posture or in any other position that is comfortable. The most important thing is to keep your back straight to prevent yourself from becoming sleepy.
- Close your eyes and turn your attention to your breathing. Breathe naturally, preferably through your nostrils, without attempting to control your breath.
- Become aware of the sensation of the breath as it enters and leaves your nostrils. This sensation is your object of meditation. Try to concentrate on it to the exclusion of everything else.
- There will be a great temptation to follow the different thoughts as they arise, but instead try to remain focused on the sensation of the breath.
- If you discover that your mind has wandered and is following your thoughts, you should return it to the breath.
- Repeat this as many times as necessary until the mind settles on the breath.

---

## Mental Rehearsal

*Mental Rehearsal* is a visualisation process in which you mentally rehearse the way you would like to think, feel and behave during a future event. *Mental Rehearsal* refers to using your mind to 'replicate the experience of the actual doing of the thing'. *Mental Rehearsal* can be used to rehearse new behaviours and future successes.

*How to do Mental Rehearsal*

- Take some time to settle down and relax.
- Enter a hypnotic state.
- Begin to imagine the future as you would like to experience it.
- Use all of your senses so that you are imagining this event as if it was happening now.
- Pay attention to the details as you rehearse the new behaviour or future success.
- Practise this new behaviour/success by repeating the event a few times.

- Try to do this *Mental Rehearsal* twice a day; it may take anything from five to thirty minutes.

## *Creative Tasks*

A *Creative Task* can be any creative activity that will facilitate insight or change. *Creative Tasks* can help us access the wisdom and resourcefulness of the unconscious mind. Creating a collage is a good example of a *Creative Task* that can clarify goals and bring healing.

*How to create a collage*

- You will need: a collection of old magazines (preferably of different kinds), a big piece of cardboard (choose whatever colour is most significant for you), scissors, glue and some good music to listen to.
- Set aside plenty of time and create a space in your house where you can put your favourite music on and spread your things out and make as much mess as you like.
- Before you begin, take five to ten minutes to relax deeply and access a trance state.
- Then ask your higher self/unconscious mind, the following question: what will it be like for me when _____ (insert the goal, for example: I am in a fertile state)?
- Simply ask the question; there is no need to try to answer it. Just ask the question and then let yourself relax more deeply.
- Then, when you are ready, let your eyes open, and start going through the magazines, tearing out all the pictures, colours and words that seem to answer that question for you. You don't need to think about it, just go through the magazines quite quickly and just rip and tear anything that strikes you as being very _____ (e.g. fertile).
- When you have torn out a collection/selection of pictures, colours and words, you can then stick them down on the board as a collage. You may also like to add a photograph of yourself, or of significant others that you feel helps to answer this question.
- There is no right or wrong. Play and have fun with this.

## *Gratitudes*

Naming and identifying all the things that you are grateful for can be profoundly healing. Saying *Gratitudes* on a daily basis helps maintain perspective. It releases endorphins, increases feelings of wellbeing and creates a new focus of attention.

*How to do Gratitudes*

- Start every day by saying 21 things that you are grateful for in your life, for example: Thank you for my healthy body; thank you for all the people I have in my life who love me; thank you for the sunshine today …

or

- Keep a journal; and every day write down three:
    - Things that happened that you are grateful for
    - Qualities in you that made those things possible
    - Actions that you took to make those things possible.

---

## *Menstrual Diary*

A *Menstrual Diary* is a notebook in which you keep track of your menstrual cycle and make note of mental, emotional and physical changes. This can be useful for developing a deeper awareness of your cycle, charting fertile times, noting premenstrual symptoms etc.

*How to keep a Menstrual Diary*

- Choose a notebook that you like.
- Create a new entry each day.
- Include information that will be useful for you, such as:
    - Date
    - Day of your cycle (Day 1 is the first day of your period)
    - Thoughts
    - Feelings
    - Physical sensations
    - Symptoms.

## 7:11 Breathing

The *7:11 Breathing* exercise takes its name from the length of the inhalation and exhalation. A wide variety of breathing exercises can be useful. The importance of this technique is its emphasis on extending the exhalation which will increase relaxation and help balance the autonomic nervous system. Breathing is a very effective self-help tool that can create a feeling of relaxation and increased wellbeing.

*How to do the 7:11 Breathing*

- Place your hands on your diaphragm which is located underneath the bottom of your ribcage.
- Inhale through your nose for the count of seven.
- Pause briefly, then exhale through your mouth for the count of 11.
- Feel your hands moving towards each other as you exhale.
- Repeat a few times until you feel more relaxed.

---

## Quick Body Scan

A *Quick Body Scan* can be done several times throughout the day. Regular body scans get you to notice and release tension in your body and help you to become more attuned to what your body needs. Body scans can help increase overall levels of mental and physical relaxation.

*How to practise body awareness throughout the day*

- While you are going about your normal activities, try to scan your body as often as possible.
- Notice how you are feeling.
- Notice where you are holding tension, and use your breath to release it.

or

- When you do daily *Self-Hypnosis* use it as a time to give your attention to your body and the sensations that are present. Imagine looking at your bodily sensations through a zoom lens and listen to any messages your body has for you.

## Emotional Bank Account

The *Emotional Bank Account* can be used to gauge and measure your state of wellbeing on a day-to-day basis. You can take greater responsibility for and manage your overall wellbeing because the *Emotional Bank Account* keeps track of all the 'expenses' or 'debits' (all the things that drain, tire and deplete you) and all the 'deposits' or 'credits' (all the things that nurture, nourish, rejuvenate you and leave you feeling good) that you make on a daily basis.

Keeping your *Emotional Bank Account* in credit will give you the resources, reserves and energy that you need to deal with things more easily in your daily life.

*How to manage your Emotional Bank Account*

- At the end of each day, make a note of all the events or activities that were debits from your account.
- Make a note of all the events or activities that were credits to your account.
- Compare the amount of credits and debits on your account for the day.
- If your account is in debit at the end of the day, decide what you will do within the next 36 hours to bring your account back into balance.

---

## Nurturing

When you nurture yourself you feel better, and your self-esteem and health improve. Self-nurturing is part of the process and preparation for parenthood.

*How to Nurture yourself*

- Start by giving yourself permission to take time for yourself
- Find ways to nurture yourself for 30 minutes each day
- Take an afternoon nap
- Have a massage
- Go for a gentle walk in nature
- Read a book
- Listen to your favourite music
- Sit in the garden with your favourite magazine

Self-nurturing should never feel like a chore. It should be something you look forward to doing.

---

## *Cognitive Restructuring*

*Cognitive Restructuring* helps you free yourself from destructive thought patterns by putting negative beliefs to the test.

*How to challenge negative thoughts when you're experiencing emotional disturbance*

1. First, become aware of and identify the negative thought. Then ask yourself the following questions:
2. Does this thought contribute to my stress?
3. Where did I learn this thought?
4. Is this thought logical?
5. Is this thought true?
6. What would I prefer to think that would allow me to feel better?

*Example*

The following example uses a very typical unhealthy belief. Below it is an example of how someone could go about challenging this belief by using the questions above.

> If I can't have a biological child I am a failure.

1. This makes me feel as if the success and happiness of my entire life depends on this one single thing, thus contributing to my stress.
2. My family does not respect my career and places a very high value on producing and raising children. My husband thinks that if your children are not your own, then there is no point having any.
3. This is not logical. All people have worth and value whether they produce children or not. Worth is determined by our actions and not by whether we produce genetic offspring.
4. This thought isn't true. Firstly I am going to do everything in my power to conceive. Then if I can't conceive I will consider other paths to

parenthood. I can be a successful and happy person whether I give birth, adopt a child or choose to remain childless.
5. I now create a new thought that will allow me to feel better: I am going to try my best to conceive but if I don't, I will find other ways to make my dreams come true and become a success.

(Domar, 2002, p. 65)

## Self-Talk SUDS

A SUDS (Subjective Units of Disturbance Scale) can be used as a way to gauge and quantify one's own level of disturbance. This is typically done on a scale of 0 to 10 where 10 represents the greatest level of disturbance and 0 represents no disturbance at all. Once the disturbance has been gauged, you can then use the scale to determine how your self-talk would need to change in order to reduce the level of disturbance on the scale.

*How to use the Self-Talk SUDS*

- Notice when you feel disturbed and become aware of what you are saying to yourself, for example, 'If this treatment fails it would be the worst thing ever …'
- Rate your level of disturbance on the SUDS where 10 is the worst it could be and 0 represents no disturbance at all.
- Ask yourself: 'What would I need to tell myself in order to bring that anxiety down on the scale?' For example, 'I really don't know what the outcome will be and right now I am doing everything I can to give it a good shot of working …'
- When you have identified this statement, say it to yourself and notice how your rating goes down on the scale.

# *Polarity Exercise*

The *Polarity Exercise* helps you challenge your fears and unhealthy beliefs by voicing both the 'best case' and 'worst case' scenarios. Doing this will reduce anxiety and restore a sense of choice and control.

*How to do the Polarity Exercise*

This exercise can be done before or during a problem situation. For example, if you have been feeling anxious about meeting with your doctor or consultant you may choose to do it before you see them.

- Notice what you are telling yourself about the situation that is creating the anxiety.
- What is the worst case scenario?
- What is the best case scenario?
- Use the answers to these questions to fill in the _____. Say it out loud to yourself.
- I allow myself to be _____ (insert the worst case scenario) and I very much look forward to it.
    - I allow myself to feel completely nervous, anxious and out of control when I am talking to the doctor… and I very much look forward to it …
- I also allow myself to be _____ (insert the best case scenario) and I very much look forward to it.
    - I also allow myself to feel totally calm and at ease with myself no matter what happens … and I very much look forward to it …
- Repeat these two opposing statements three times.

# Section D: Paths To Parenthood

If you are working with fertility problems you need to understand the different paths to parenthood so that you can support your client, irrespective of how they choose to pursue parenthood.

In this section we will look at the different options available, including natural conception, assisted fertility, surrogacy, adoption and fostering. I have provided some basic information about the different options and some useful information about the physiology of natural conception.

You will find descriptions of the different medical treatments that are currently available as well as detailed treatment plans for supporting assisted reproductive treatments such as IVF.

**This section contains:**

**Paths to parenthood**
- Natural conception .................................................................................296
- Assisted fertility treatments ...................................................................297
- Surrogacy ..................................................................................................298
- Adoption ...................................................................................................298
- Fostering ...................................................................................................299

**Things you may need to know about natural conception**
- The menstrual cycle ................................................................................300
- How to determine the fertile time .......................................................304
- The male reproductive system ..............................................................305
- Human development: conception to birth ........................................305

**Assisted Reproductive Technology (ART)**
- Introduction to ART ...............................................................................309
- Medical treatments .................................................................................310
- Sucess rates for ART ...............................................................................316
- The positive impact of mind-body approaches on ART ..................317
- The *Fertile Body Method* for ART ......................................................320
- The 3 Session Plan For ART ..................................................................321
- The *Fertile Body Method* and IVF .....................................................330
- The 4 Session Plan For IVF ...................................................................332
- The Complete Plan For IVF ..................................................................344
- Adapting the IVF plan for egg, sperm and embryo donation ........346

## *Paths to parenthood*

There are many different paths to parenthood. It may be useful to inform your client about the different options available to them. Sometimes just knowing that there are other options can help couples maintain hope. While most couples would prefer to have children of their own, they often find it comforting to know that even if they can't have their own biological children, they may still be able to become parents. If your client is aware of all the options for parenthood before they start assisted fertility treatments, this means that possible treatment failure can be handled more easily.

Below I have included a short description of each path to parenthood and provided some basic information about each option. This information may be useful in discussing the different options with your client or for understanding more about the path your client has chosen. I would recommend that you refer your client to relevant experts to discuss their options in more detail and to answer any questions they may have.

I feel that my role as role as a practitioner of the *Fertile Body Method* is to draw the client's attention to the options available to them and to help them to explore their attitudes and feelings about these possibilities. I can also support them in making decisions about which avenue to pursue.

The decision-making process can be very difficult for some couples because they feel that the risk of making the 'wrong' decision is high. Some women fear that they may live to regret their decision and spend the rest of their life wishing that they had done something different.

## *Natural conception*

As we all know, natural conception occurs as a result of sexual intercourse that takes place during the woman's fertile time. The exact moment of fertilisation is when a woman's egg and a man's sperm fuse to form a single cell. But for this to happen successfully, certain things must be in place. The systems of the body that are involved in the production of eggs and sperm must be working optimally. In addition, intercourse must take place around the time of ovulation when an egg has been released from the ovary.

*Case study: difficult decisions*

A client who came to see me after trying to conceive unsuccessfully for a year felt very opposed to IVF treatment. She had been diagnosed with unexplained infertility and was adamant that she did not want to go down the IVF route. While she was sure that she did not want to go for assisted medical treatment, she also felt anxious about making the decision. When we explored this further, she realised that she felt most anxious about not having a baby and it being her 'fault' because she had chosen not to have IVF. She wanted to feel confident that she was making the 'right' decision. We spent some time looking at why she felt so opposed to IVF and how she knew she wanted to conceive naturally. For homework I asked her to write down all the reasons she had for choosing not to do IVF, as well as all the reasons she had for choosing natural conception. I also suggested that she discuss this more fully with her husband, who also felt strongly about not pursuing IVF.

*Parts Work* helped her access the inner resources that she needed to feel at peace with her decision, irrespective of whether she had children or not. I also pseudo-orientated her into a future time where she was able to see how this inner resource would support her in her decision, even if she had not conceived naturally. Her anxiety about living to regret her decision diminished and she felt free to focus her attention on the things that she could do to improve her chances of natural conception.

## Assisted fertility treatments

Assisted fertility treatments are available to couples who have had problems conceiving naturally. These treatments include fertility drugs, IUI (intra-uterine insemination), GIFT (gamete intra-Fallopian transfer), IVF (in vitro fertilisation) and ICSI (intra-cytoplasmic sperm injection). Donated eggs and/or sperm are also an option for those who do not have healthy, viable eggs or sperm.

More information about these treatments and how to work with people undergoing them is available in the *Assisted Reproductive Technology* section (Page 308).

## Surrogacy

- A surrogate carries and gives birth to a baby for another woman. There are two types of surrogacy – straight and host surrogacy.

- Straight surrogacy means that the surrogate uses her own egg and fertilises it with the intended father's sperm.

- Host surrogacy uses the father's sperm fertilised with the mother's egg, and is implanted into the surrogate using IVF.

- For further information, go to www.surrogacy.org.uk.

Surrogacy may be an option if:

- The woman has a medical condition that makes it impossible or dangerous for her to get pregnant and give birth.

- The couple have been unsuccessful with IVF.

## Adoption

Adoption is the legal act of permanently placing a child with a parent or parents other than the birth (or 'biological', or 'natural') mother or father.

People who have fertility problems may find it helpful to learn as much as possible about adoption so that they can think about whether or not it is a possible option for them. After years of difficult treatment, some people may feel that adoption is a simple solution. Other may decide that adoption is a last resort, or possibly that it is not an option at all.

When a couple has decided to adopt they will be told to wait six months after ending fertility treatment before applying. This wait is suggested to encourage people to integrate their past experiences and grieve the loss of not being biological parents.

Encourage the client to make use of this time by learning more about adoption issues, attending adoption information evenings and giving themselves time to grieve and come to terms with what they have been through. They may need support and help to feel truly ready to go ahead with adopting.

For further information about adoption, go to www.adoption.org.uk.

## Fostering

Fostering is a way of providing family life for someone else's child in your own home when they are unable to live with their birth family. This can be due to many reasons: illness, relationship problems, family breakdown, or perhaps a situation where the child's welfare is threatened.

Fostering differs from adoption in that an adoption order ends a child's legal relationship with their natural family, whereas fostered children remain the legal responsibility of the local authority and/or their birth parents.

Foster carers provide a safe, secure and stable environment for these children and young people and the foster care placement can last for days, months or even years. Many children return home to their families, but others may receive long-term support either through continued fostering, adoption, residential care or by being helped to live independently.

For further information about fostering, go to www.fostering.org.uk.

## *Things you may need to know about natural conception*

Most people working in this field will already have a good understanding of the physiology of natural conception. For those who are new to this field, the information below will provide you with a basic understanding of what you need to know to work accurately and confidently with natural conception.

I have found that having an understanding of the physiology of conception has allowed me to help people connect with their bodies and have a better understanding of how they can support and enhance their fertility.

### *The menstrual cycle*

If a woman understands her menstrual cycle and pays close attention to it, she can become more conscious of the effects these changes are having on her, psychologically and emotionally. This awareness can empower and help women to take positive steps so that they may support themselves throughout their cycle. Understanding the cycle and learning to work with it instead of against it can also resolve menstrual health problems. I have included more information about how to create menstrual health in *Stage 3: Resolve* (Page 115). The information provided below is intended to support this work by giving you a biological understanding of the menstrual cycle and fertility.

Despite being one of the most common events in the lives of half the population, the menstrual cycle is still one of the most widely misunderstood biological functions and is subject to more myths and misconceptions than perhaps any other area of human physiology. Furthermore, many cultural attitudes, beliefs and ongoing myths mean that menstruation is a little talked-about subject. The following information should provide you with a basic understanding of menstruation and fertility awareness. For more detailed information on fertility indicators refer to the Fertility Awareness Education programme and the recommended reading list in the Resources section (Page 351).

The menstrual cycle can be divided into two stages:

i. The follicular phase: menstruation to ovulation.
ii. The luteal phase: ovulation to menstruation.

The length of a woman's menstrual cycle is calculated by the number of days between one period and the next. A cycle begins on the first day of bleeding and continues up to, but not including, the first day of the next period. Women's cycles range from 21 to 40 days or more, with an average of about 28 days. The length of a woman's cycle may change a little or a lot from month to month. In a healthy cycle ovulation occurs 12 to 16 days prior to menstruation irrespective of whether a woman's cycle is short or long. Menstruation can last from one to eight days, with the average being four to five days.

*The follicular phase: menstruation to ovulation*

> This stage begins with menstruation and can vary greatly in length. It may last anywhere between 6 and 21 days. Women in this phase are considered semi or partly fertile because there is no way of knowing how many days it will be until ovulation.
>
> The first day of bleeding is day one of the menstrual cycle. Bleeding will start when oestrogen and progesterone levels in a woman's body are at their lowest causing the lining of the womb to start to shed.
>
> At about the same time the hypothalamus starts producing gonadotrophin-releasing hormone (GnRH) which stimulates a small gland at the base of the brain, the pituitary, to release follicle stimulating hormone (FSH). This in turn triggers about 10 to 20 follicles, or egg sacs, to start developing in the ovaries. Only one, sometimes two, of these will mature fully.
>
> The developing follicles produce oestrogen and as oestrogen levels rise, the following changes occur:
>
> - The endometrium (lining of the uterus) becomes thicker in preparation for a fertilised egg.
> - The cervix becomes higher, softer and more open.
> - Cervical mucus produced by the glands in the cervix changes to a 'sperm-friendly' mucus.
> - The volume of fluid mucus increases.
> - Highly fertile mucus is 98% water. It appears transparent, glistening, slippery and stretchy.
> - The basal body temperature remains at a lower level.
>
> Once the oestrogen produced by the growing follicles reaches a certain level, it triggers the pituitary gland to release a surge of LH (luteinising hormone). This causes the most mature follicle to burst open and release its egg into the Fallopian tube. This is ovulation.
>
> Some women feel a slight twinge on one side of their lower back or abdominal area around the time of ovulation. Not every woman experiences

this, but it is normal and is known as mittelschmerz (middle pain). Some women may also have discharge that is pinkish or a little bloody.

*The luteal phase: ovulation to menstruation*

This phase lasts from ovulation to menstruation and it is generally accepted that it is always 12 to 16 days long, whether the cycle is short, average or long.

After the egg has been released at ovulation, the remains of the egg sac forms a small yellow body called the corpus luteum, which then starts producing the hormone progesterone. The increased levels of progesterone cause the following changes to occur:

- The blood supply to the lining of the womb increases.
- The endometrium softens in preparation for the implantation of a fertilised ovum.
- The cervix becomes lower, firmer and closed.
- Cervical mucus becomes hostile, preventing sperm penetration.
- After ovulation there is a rapid return to the infertile state. A dense network of filaments forms a thick, sticky mucus plug that impedes sperm penetration. Sperm are rapidly destroyed by the acidic vaginal secretions.
- The basal body temperature is raised by about 0.2°C or more.

The egg is normally fertilised in the Fallopian tube and will take about five days to reach the womb. By the time it embeds itself in the womb lining, it will be made up of about 150 cells. The corpus luteum will continue to produce progesterone to nourish the fertilised egg.

If fertilisation does not occur, the corpus luteum will remain for about fourteen days and then shrivel and die, causing progesterone levels to plummet. As a result, the blood vessels in the womb lining break up, the walls of the womb contract and the lining of the womb sheds. This is the beginning of menstruation.

*Paths to Parenthood*

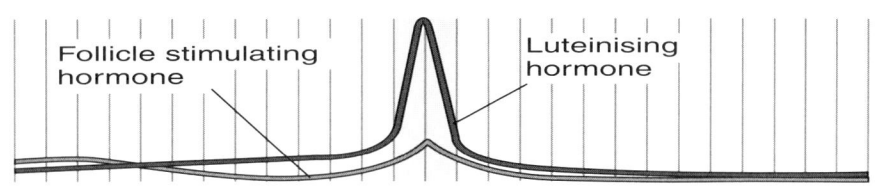

**Pituitary Hormone Cycle**
- Follicle stimulating hormone
- Luteinising hormone

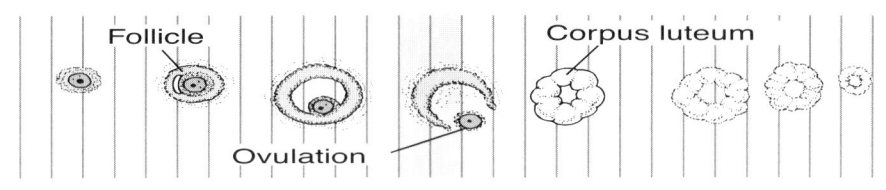

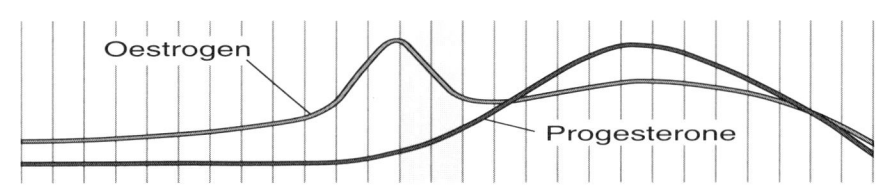

**Ovarian Cycle**
- Follicle
- Ovulation
- Corpus luteum

**Sex Hormone Cycle**
- Oestrogen
- Progesterone

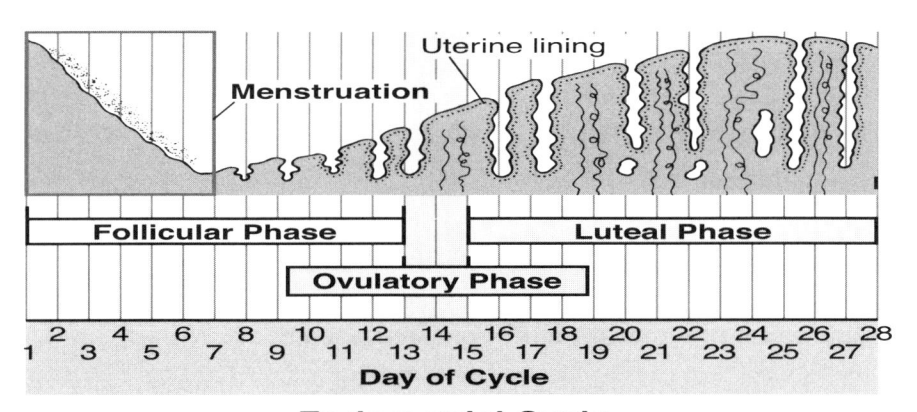

**Endometrial Cycle**
- Menstruation
- Uterine lining
- Follicular Phase
- Ovulatory Phase
- Luteal Phase
- Day of Cycle

*Diagram showing the changes that occur during the menstrual cycle*
[Diagrams from http://www.merck.com/mmhe/sec22/ch241/ch241e.html]

The Fertile Body Method

## How to determine the fertile time

A man is always potentially fertile, whereas a woman's fertility works on a cyclical basis. The few days leading up to ovulation are considered the most fertile in a woman's cycle. Sperm can survive for up to five days in a woman's body but on average they live for three days. If a woman has sex or insemination during the five or six days before she ovulates, it is likely that the sperm will still be around by the time her egg is released. One or two days after ovulation are also considered fertile days because a woman's egg can live for about 20 hours after ovulation. If two eggs have matured, the second will be released within 24 hours of the first. From a few days after ovulation until her next bleed, a woman is generally not fertile.

Every woman's fertility pattern is unique and may vary from month to month. A woman can learn to identify her fertile times by observing physiological changes in her body, using a combination of indicators of fertility. These indicators are scientifically proven to reflect changes in the ovarian hormone levels and to predict fertility status accurately.

### Indicators of fertility

- Waking temperature: basal body temperature (BBT)
- Cervical mucus changes
- Changes in the cervix
- Calculation of cycle length
- Abdominal pain and breast symptoms (minor indicators).

For more detailed information on fertility indicators refer to the Fertility Awareness Education programme in the Resources section.

### Other ways to determine ovulation

- Ovulation predictor kits measure the amount of luteinising hormone (LH) found in the urine. A LH surge occurs 24 to 36 hours before ovulation. There are some cases in which these tests will be inaccurate.

- Saliva tests measure the salt content in the saliva. Salt levels rise as oestrogen levels increase (increased oestrogen is a sign that ovulation is about to occur). This method tends to have a high level of accuracy.

## The male reproductive system

The primary hormones involved in the male reproductive system are follicle-stimulating hormone, luteinising hormone, gonadotrophin-releasing hormone and testosterone.

Gonadotrophin-releasing hormone, or GnRH, produced by the hypothalamus in the brain, triggers the release of follicle-stimulating hormone (FSH) and luteinising hormone (LH) from the pituitary gland. FSH stimulates sperm production in the testicles while LH stimulates the testicles to produce testosterone.

From the testicles, sperm travel to the epididymis, a 12m-long coiled tube, where they mature, which takes between nine and ten weeks. It takes seventy days for a new sperm to develop into a mature swimmer, so the lifestyle changes that a man makes today will show themselves in two to three months time.

The mature sperm then travel down another tube, the vas deferens, to the penis, ready for their next journey. At the point of ejaculation during intercourse, the penis releases as many as 300 million sperm into the woman's vagina but only a few survive the hazardous journey through the neck of the womb, uterus and Fallopian tubes.

The tip of the sperm head is called the acrosome, which enables the sperm to penetrate the egg. The mid-piece contains the mitochondria, which supplies the energy the tail needs to move. The tail's whip-like movements propel the sperm towards the egg. Ultimately, only one sperm will burrow its way into the egg.

The head of the sperm contains the DNA, which when combined with the egg's DNA, will create a unique individual.

## Human development: conception to birth

There are five stages in the development of a human being, starting from conception and ending in birth. I have used this information in my own practice to create accurate, detailed and engaging guided visualisations for clients. The *Conception* script in Section C (Page 276) is an example a guided visualisation using the five stages of development to help women envisage a successful conception and implantation.

*The five stages of development*

1. Human development starts at the moment of conception when the sperm penetrates the egg and they combine to form a zygote. The zygote contains all the necessary genetic information from the sperm and egg. Tiny hair-like cilia lining the Fallopian tube propel the zygote through the tube toward the uterus. The zygote's cells divide repeatedly as it moves down the Fallopian tube. The journey takes three to five days. In the uterus, the cells continue to divide, becoming a hollow ball of cells called a blastocyst.

2. The blastocyst consists of an inner group of cells with an outer shell. The inner group of cells will become the embryo, while the outer group of cells will become the placenta. The placenta produces several hormones that help maintain the pregnancy. It also carries oxygen and nutrients from the mother to the foetus and waste materials from the foetus to the mother. Five to eight days after fertilisation the blastocyst attaches to the womb lining and begins to implant into the uterine wall. At this point the lining of the uterus has grown and is ready to support the foetus. The blastocyst sticks tightly to the lining, where it receives nourishment via the mother's bloodstream.

3. During the third stage of development the embryo begins to form. The cells of the embryo now multiply and begin to take on specific functions. This process is called differentiation and leads to the various cell types that make up a human being (such as blood cells, kidney cells, and nerve cells). There is rapid growth, and the baby's main external features begin to take form.

4. The end of the eighth week marks the end of the embryonic stage and the beginning of the foetal stage, which lasts until birth. During this time, the structures that have already formed continue to grow and develop. By 12 weeks of pregnancy the foetus fills the entire uterus and its heartbeat can be heard. As the placenta develops, it extends tiny hair-like villi into the wall of the uterus. The villi branch out to form an intricate, tree-like structure that increases the area of contact between the wall of the uterus and the placenta, so that more nutrients and waste materials can be exchanged. The placenta is fully formed by 18 to 20 weeks but continues to grow throughout pregnancy. At delivery, it weighs about one pound.

5. The fifth and final stage is the birth itself.

*Paths to Parenthood*

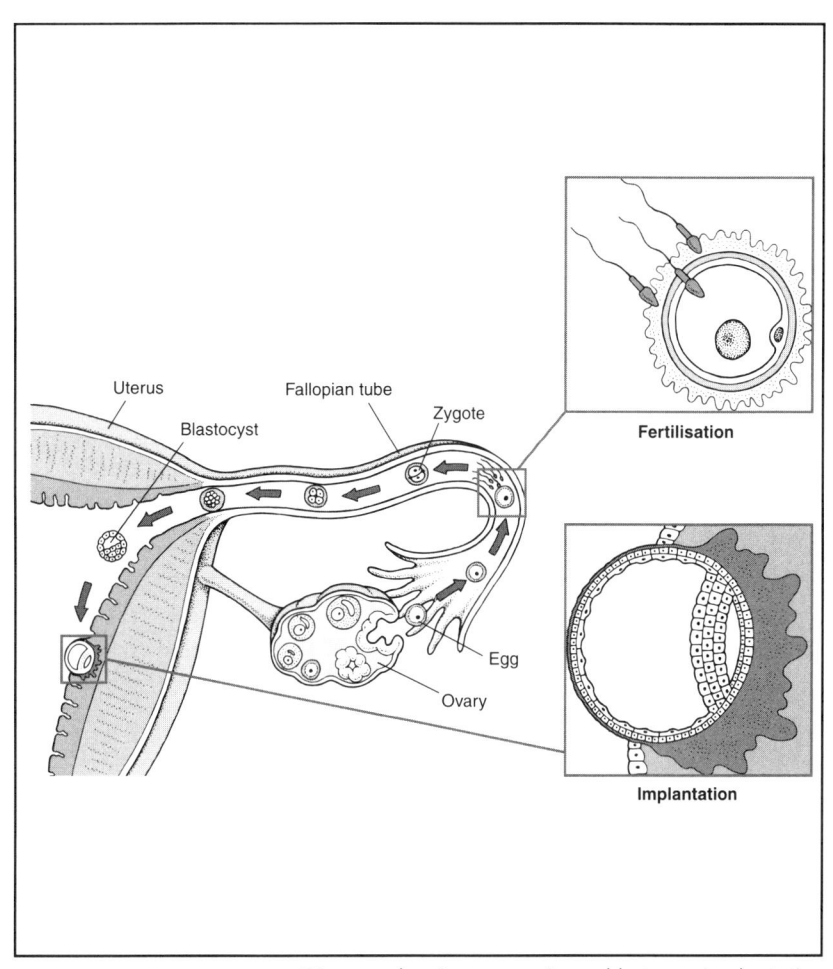

*Diagram showing conception to blastocyst implantation*

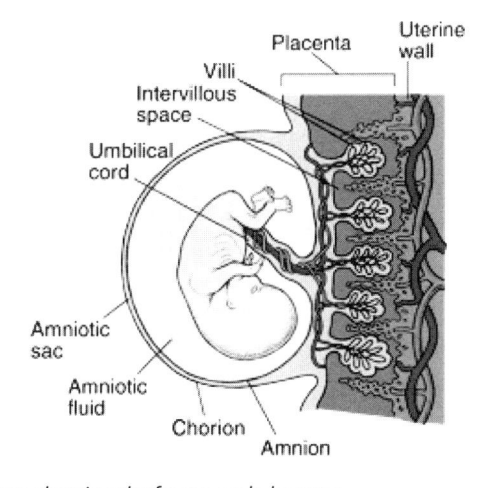

*Diagram showing the foetus and placenta*

## Assisted Reproductive Technology (ART)

This section contains information about Assisted Reproductive Technology and how the *Fertile Body Method* can help women who are undergoing fertility treatment. It covers the different medical treatments available and includes some interesting research about the positive impact of mind-body approaches on ART.

This section addresses women specifically, because they are usually more directly involved in the medical intervention. It is possible that men may come to see you about issues related to fertility, such as sexual performance anxiety or poor sperm motility; the information provided in Section B (Page 23) addresses this.

The *Fertile Body Method* includes three treatment plans for ART. The first treatment plan can be used with any type of ART and the second two plans are for IVF specifically. Each treatment plan is outlined and described, and suggestions for useful scripts, techniques and self-help tools are included. For a full description of these techniques and tools please refer to Section C (Page 181).

The three treatment plans offer a guide for structuring your therapeutic approach and can be applied and adapted according to your client's specific needs. Case studies for each plan illustrate a possible way in which you might apply the structure.

This section contains:

- Introduction to ART
- Current medical treatments available
- The positive impact of mind-body approaches on ART
- The *Fertile Body Method* for ART
- The 3 Session Plan For ART
- *The Fertile Body Method* and IVF
- The 4 Session Plan For IVF
- The Complete Plan For IVF
- Adapting the IVF plan for egg, sperm and embryo donation.

## Introduction to ART

Medical technology is developing rapidly and the types of fertility treatments available are continuing to evolve and change. It is important for therapists to understand what the current treatments are and how they work – this will help you formulate appropriate and relevant sessions. Therapy will be most valuable for people going through ART if the sessions are tailored to work alongside the medical treatment.

It is also important for you to be familiar with the names of different treatments, as well as some of the medical terminology. I have often been amazed at how much the women I work with know about the medical aspects of their fertility treatment. Many of them are able to rattle off the names of drugs, dosages and hormone levels as if they had a degree in reproductive medicine. While it is not our role to be experts in the medical aspects of fertility treatments, it is important to understand what they are going through.

> ### Case study: medicalisation of treatment
>
> I recall an early case in my work where the client, Sari, had a spectacular understanding of the medical aspects of fertility. She had been going through fertility treatments for a number of years and made it her business to ask lots of questions. Her relationship with her own fertility had become very technical and medical. Communicating and developing rapport would have been considerably easier had I known a little bit more about the medical side.
>
> When I asked Sari about what a fertile state would be like for her, she described it as some kind of formula made up of numbers and unpronounceable words. I felt it was really important to help reconnect her with her natural fertility. She experienced a significant shift in thinking when I asked her to remember back to a time before all of these treatments had begun and to let herself forget everything that had occurred since then. Once she had accessed a pleasant memory from that time I asked her to describe what she believed a fertile state would be like for her. She became very emotionally moved and described this fertile state as being very still, soft and intimately connected with her body. She experienced it as a loving feeling, rather than a formula. At the following session she told me that for the first time since she had begun all the medical treatment, she felt strong and empowered. I asked Sari what she thought had made the difference. She said that up until now she had felt powerless because she didn't know how to make her body have the hormone levels that she needed, but she did know how to feel love and be still and intimate with her body.

> I learnt a lot from this case about the importance of understanding the medical aspects of fertility as well as the benefits of helping woman like Sari to reconnect with their innate understanding of fertility.

## *Medical treatments*

- Surgery
- Fertility drugs
- Intra-uterine insemination (IUI) or intra-cervical insemination (ICI)
- Surrogacy
- Egg, sperm or embryo donation
- In vitro fertilisation (IVF), gamete intra-Fallopian transfer (GIFT) and intra-cytoplasmic sperm injection (ICSI).

The protocols used for each treatment may vary from clinic to clinic and may also vary depending on the client's circumstances. This section gives you a basic understanding of these treatments and their terminology, along with some of the potential issues that may need to be addressed in therapy.

### Surgery

Surgery may resolve some cases of infertility by addressing the physical factors that affect conception and pregnancy. Hypnosis can be used to help the client go into the surgery feeling calm and relaxed, as well as to help increase post-operative recovery.

Who could surgery help?

- Women with blocked fallopian tubes
- Women with endometriosis
- Women with fibroids

- Women who have been sterilised
- Men who have had a vasectomy
- Men with varicocele.

*Fertility drugs*

There are many different types of fertility drugs that are designed to induce egg production and ovulation. Sometimes fertility drugs are used to aid natural conception, but usually they're used in conjunction with other medical treatments such as IUI and IVF. For IVF treatments, women are sometimes initially prescribed drugs which suppress their menstrual cycle. Drugs that help to maintain pregnancy by thickening the lining of the womb can also be given to women as part of IVF treatment.

Who is this treatment for?

- Couples undergoing medical procedures such as IUI, ICI, ICSI, GIFT and IVF
- Women who are not ovulating
- Women who have had recurrent miscarriage
- Women with irregular periods.

All fertility drugs have potential side effects that vary from drug to drug, but typically include symptoms such as:

- Hot flushes
- Night sweats
- Mood swings
- Nausea
- Breast tenderness
- Insomnia
- Headaches

- Sore muscles
- Spots and acne.

## IUI / ICI

This is a treatment in which sperm is inserted into the womb during ovulation. Some women may be prescribed fertility drugs, in the form of injections or nasal spray, to stimulate ovulation. Sperm which have been sorted and carefully selected are inserted through the cervix using a catheter.

Who is this treatment for?

- Women trying for a baby using donated sperm.
- Couples where the man has reduced sperm count or poor sperm motility.
- Women who are producing hostile cervical mucus or antibodies that prevent the sperm from surviving the journey to the womb.
- Couples who have sexual problems such as impotence or premature ejaculation.
- Unexplained infertility.

The stages of IUI/ICI treatment:

- Egg production
  - Eggs can be produced naturally or using stimulation drugs.
  - Egg development is tracked by vaginal ultrasound scans.
- Insemination and implantation
  - Insemination is done using a speculum and catheter. Please note that this may be an issue for women suffering from vaginismus, the involuntary tightening of the vaginal tract.
  - After the insemination the woman is given time to rest before returning home.
- Pregnancy test
  - The pregnancy test may be done at home or at the clinic.

## Surrogacy

Straight surrogacy uses IUI to impregnate the surrogate mother with the male partner's sperm. Host surrogacy uses IVF with the couple to produce a fertilised embryo which is then transferred into the surrogate's womb. There are other variations of surrogacy that include the use of donated eggs and/or donated sperm.

Who is this treatment for?

- Couples who have medical problems that make it dangerous or impossible to get pregnant or give birth.
- Couples who have had failed IVF treatment.

Some issues that may need to be addressed:

- How do both partners feel about surrogacy?
- What will they tell their child?
- How will they deal with the surrogate changing her mind?

## Using donated eggs, sperm or embryos

Donated eggs, sperm or embryos can be used in fertility treatments:

- Donated sperm is used in conjunction with IUI treatment.
- Donated eggs are collected from the donor and fertilised with the male partner's sperm. The fertilised embryos are then transferred into the woman's womb after fertility drugs have been taken to prepare her womb lining.
- Donated embryos can be transferred into the woman's womb in the same way, or the donated embryos can be transferred to a surrogate.

Who are these treatment options for?

- Men who are producing little or no sperm
- Men who have had a vasectomy

- Men who have poor-quality sperm
- Single mothers
- Same sex couples
- Women who have been through early menopause
- Women who have no ovaries or have low egg quality
- Women who have had recurrent miscarriages
- Women with irregular periods
- Couples who have a high risk of passing on an inherited disorder.

Some issues that may need to be addressed:

- How does the woman feel about using donated sperm, eggs or embryos?
- How does the man feels about using donated sperm, eggs or embryos?
- What will they tell the child?
- What are their concerns?

*IVF, ICSI and GIFT*

IVF
In vitro fertilisation (IVF) is a process by which egg cells are fertilised by sperm outside the woman's womb, in vitro (meaning literally, 'within a glass' or test tube). The process involves hormonally controlling the ovulatory process, removing ova (eggs) from the woman's ovaries and letting sperm fertilise them in a fluid medium. The fertilised egg (zygote) is then transferred to the womb so that implantation can occur. Pregnancy will result if the implantation is successful.

Who is this treatment for?

- Women with blocked or damaged Fallopian tubes
- Men with mild sperm problems such as reduced sperm motility
- Couples who have tried fertility drugs or IUI without success

- Couples with unexplained infertility.

## ICSI

Intra-cytoplasmic sperm injection (ICSI) is not a treatment in itself, but is used in conjunction with IVF. ICSI involves injecting a single sperm into the centre of an egg, giving it the best chance of fertilisation.

Who is this treatment for?

- Men who have a very low sperm count

- Men who have sperm abnormalities

- Women who produce few eggs during stimulation that seem capable of being fertilised.

## GIFT

Gamete intra-Fallopian transfer (GIFT) is very similar to IVF except that fertilisation happens inside the body. Once the eggs and sperm have been collected and screened, the healthiest egg/s and sperm are selected and transferred into a Fallopian tube where conception can occur naturally.

Who is this treatment for?

- Men with low sperm count

- Men with poor sperm motility

- Unexplained infertility.

Some negative side effects of IVF treatment:

- Symptomatic reaction to the drugs: includes hot flushes, night sweats, mood swings, low mood, spots and acne, irritability, vaginal dryness, headaches, restlessness, sore muscles, nausea, vomiting.

- Ovarian hyperstimulation syndrome (OHSS): a potentially dangerous reaction to the drugs used to stimulate egg production. The over stimulation can result in ovarian cysts, fluid build-up in the stomach and chest cavity, blood clots and reduced blood flow to the kidneys.

- Increased risk of multiple births: if more than one embryo is placed in the uterus there is an increased chance that multiple embryos may implant.

It's important to know about the negative side effects for two reasons: firstly, it helps you understand what your client may be experiencing; secondly, and most importantly, I hope that it will remind you always to include safety measures in your work. For example, suggestions or visualisations for the stimulation of egg production should always be combined with a suggestion such as *'your body can respond just the right amount to the stimulation.'* As seen with OHSS, if the body responds 'too well' it may be potentially dangerous. You can remind your client in trance that their body knows how to regulate their response to the treatment and that their body instinctively knows how to respond in a healthy way.

For example, I had one client who had been visualising her ovaries as a bunch of ripening grapes. She came to see me for her second session after a few days of taking the ovarian stimulation drugs. She had just been for a scan and told me that she had been feeling unwell but was pleased at how many follicles had already grown. Her nurse had said that there was no cause for concern at this stage so we did some work together to reduce the negative side effects she was feeling. Her insight during the trance session provided a valuable lesson and reminder to us both. When she went into the *Control Room* of her mind and body, I suggested that her attention be drawn to the controls which were responsible for the side effects she was experiencing. When she was standing in front of the controls she noticed that the dial responsible was set to the 'red setting'. On a screen in front of her she saw the image she had been visualising of a ripe bunch of grapes. As she began to turn the dial from the 'red setting' to the 'green setting' the image changed from being a big bunch of 40 ripe grapes to a smaller bunch of 9 ripe grapes. She reported feeling a release of tension in her body when she changed the dial to its optimum 'green setting'. After the session her symptoms subsided and she felt significantly better during the remainder of her IVF treatment.

## Success rates for ART

The success rates for ART are not particularly high and having medical treatment does not necessarily increase a woman's chances of conceiving. There are certain cases, specifically with unexplained infertility, where the chances of conceiving naturally are potentially higher than conceiving using IVF, so couples going for treatments such as IVF stand a significant chance that it won't work. Going into treatment knowing that you have a 70% or more chance of it failing is likely to increase feelings of desperation and levels of stress.

With these low success rates, you will always need to spend time building your clients' inner resources so that they can cope more easily with possible treatment failure.

The average success rate for IVF treatment using fresh eggs in the UK is:

- 30% for women under 35
- 24% for women aged 35 to 37
- 18% for women aged 38 to 39
- 10% for women aged 40 to 42
- 3% for women aged 43 to 44
- 1% for women aged over 44.

The average success rate for donor insemination treatment in the UK is:

- 13% for women under 35
- 10% for women aged 35 to 39
- 4% for women aged 40 to 42
- 2% for women aged 43 to 44.

Statistics from the HFEA published in conjunction with the *HFEA Guide to Infertility* treatment and success data based on treatment carried out in 2005 (HEFA, 2008).

## The positive impact of mind-body approaches on ART

The field of ART is relatively new and as yet there has not been much research carried out on the effects of mind-body approaches on medical treatment. However, the research which has been done suggests that mind-body approaches can be beneficial and when used to support fertility treatment, can increase the success rates.

James Schwartz, a hypnotherapist and NLP (neuro-linguistic Programming) practitioner in America, has compiled some of the research evidence supporting mind-body approaches for fertility. In his book *The mind-body fertility connection:*

*The true pathway to conception* (Schwartz, 2008), Schwartz cites the following examples which show the positive impact of mind-body approaches on ART:

> There have been 14 major published studies investigating how levels of distress can affect a woman's success when she undergoes an IVF cycle. Dr Alice Domar summarises the results of those studies:
>
> Ten of the studies showed that distress levels are indeed associated with decreased pregnancy rates. The more anxiety or depression the women expressed before undergoing IVF, the less likely they were to get pregnant. In several of the studies the results were dramatic; for example, in one study the most depressed women experienced half the pregnancy rates of the least depressed women. Two of the fourteen studies had small sample sizes and the results showed trends (i.e. there was a tendency for the distressed women to have lower pregnancy rates), but the results fell just short of statistical significance. Two of the studies showed no relationship between distress and pregnancy rates.
> (Domar, 2002, pp. 1–5)
>
> Philip Quinn, along with Dr Michael Pawson, published the results of their landmark study in 1994, in an article called 'Psychosomatic Infertility,' published in the European Journal of Clinical Hypnosis (Quinn and Pawson, 1994). The 'Psychosomatic Infertility' study took a group of women between the ages of 26 and 42 (with a mean age of 32) who had been infertile from two to twelve years (with a mean of three-and-a-half years), and each of those women participated in an average of nine hypnotherapy sessions. Nine of those women received additional treatments such as IVF or GIFT. Twenty-six of the forty-two women (65%) went on to have successful full-term pregnancies.

Dr Alice Domar has been one of the major researchers in mind-body medicine and fertility and her work is often referred to by hypnotherapists. In her book *Conquering Infertility*, she cites the following study that shows the effect of depression on IVF:

> Another study showed that women who had experienced at least one unsuccessful IVF cycle and who had depressive symptoms before continuing IVF treatment experienced a 13% subsequent pregnancy rate, in contrast to a 29% pregnancy rate in women who did not experience depressive symptoms before their IVF cycle.
> (Domar, 2002, p. 24)

The following study cited in *Conquering Infertility* is also of interest since it suggests that if we address some of the psychological and emotional issues in patients undergoing IVF they may be less likely to experience the negative side effects of IVF medication.

*A study done comparing IVF patients and Egg Donor patients undergoing IVF showed that there are far fewer psychological and emotional effects from the [stimulation] medication in the egg donors. This suggests that the mood swings and anxiety experienced by infertility patients is not solely as a result of the medication.*
(Domar, 2002, pp. 223–4) [IVF patients undergo stimulation in order to produce eggs for their own treatment whereas Egg Donor patients undergo stimulation in order to donate them, i.e. the Egg Donor has no emotional investment in the outcome of stimulation.]

Professor Eliahu Levitas' study, published in the *Fertility and Sterility Journal* in 2004, shows the benefit of using hypnosis during embryo transfer. Conducted by Levitas and his team at Soroka Hospital in Israel, the study aimed to determine if hypnosis could improve the success of the embryo transfers stage of IVF.

The study of 185 women found that 28% of those who were hypnotised for the IVF treatment became pregnant, compared with 14% of the women in the control group (Levitas, 2006). Professor Levitas studied the effects of hypnosis on embryo transfer because prior studies had demonstrated that the stress of the medical procedure created small contractions in the uterus that prevented the fertilised egg from successfully implanting. He indicated that tranquilisers had been used in prior studies, but nothing worked as well as hypnosis. The study showed that hypnosis effectively doubles the success of IVF treatments.

There is still a lot of scope and potential for further research on the effects of mind-body approaches on ART. The current success rates for ART are relatively low and I believe they could be significantly improved through an integrated approach.

The advances in reproductive medicine have created the possibility of parenthood for many couples who otherwise may have had no choice. However, until it is fully acknowledged that fertility is affected by a wide variety of factors, the success of treatment is unlikely to improve. Carefully selected combinations of treatments that address the couple's mental, emotional, physical and energetic health are key. I would like to encourage therapists who have an interest in research to consider doing further studies in this area. I hope that further research into mind-body approaches will make an integrated approach more mainstream.

## *The* Fertile Body Method *for ART*

The six stages of the *Fertile Body Method* can be used to support ART in much the same way as they are used to support natural conception. The way the framework is applied very much depends on the time, money and commitment your client is willing to consign to therapy.

Ideally I like to see clients a few weeks before they are due to start treatment, so that we have time to create a good *Outcome* and restore *Balance* and wellbeing (Stage 2) before their fertility treatment begins. The better the client's mental, emotional and physical state is when they undergo treatment, the more likely it is to be successful. In cases where there are pressing issues that need to be resolved (Stage 3), such as relationship problems or fears about giving birth, it would be best to address these before fertility treatment begins.

During fertility treatment, the main focus of the *Fertile Body Method* is to *Enhance* (Stage 4) and *Prepare* (Stage 5). While a lot of mental, emotional and physical preparation can be done before treatment begins, hypnosis can be very useful during treatment to help optimise the body's response to the medical interventions. Throughout the various treatment plans I will be giving suggestions of techniques and scripts that can be used to enhance the effectiveness of medical treatment and help the client prepare mentally, emotionally and physically. Visualisations that are designed to enhance and prepare the client can be repeated and reinforced through *Self-Hypnosis* or a self-hypnosis CD. An often-overlooked stage of therapy is supporting the client after they have heard the results of their treatment. Sessions after their fertility treatment results can be used to provide emotional *Support* or to maintain the changes (Stage 6) that they have made.

Many of the women I see, who would like to use hypnosis to support their medical treatment, contact me when their treatment has already begun or is about to begin. *The 3 Session Plan For ART* and *The 4 Session Plan For IVF* have evolved as a result of these clients' experiences. Others are able to undergo hypnosis well before they start medical treatment, so I have created three different approaches to suit different needs:

- *The 3 Session Plan For ART*: for supporting ART (excluding IVF) in cases where you see the client for the first time once medical treatment has already begun or is about to begin. This plan can be used to support all the various medical treatments, from fertility drugs to egg donation.

- *The 4 Session Plan For IVF*: for supporting IVF in cases where you see your client for the first time once medical treatment has already begun or is about to begin. This plan is designed specifically for supporting IVF, ICSI and GIFT treatment.

- *The Complete Plan For IVF*: an in-depth plan for supporting IVF (including ICSI and GIFT) treatment where you start seeing the client before medical treatment begins. This plan combines the six stages of the *Fertile Body Method* with *The 4 Session Plan For IVF*. The complete plan will consist of six or more sessions and is the most thorough approach for supporting and enhancing IVF.

## The 3 Session Plan For ART

This plan is suitable for clients who come for therapy when their fertility treatment is already under way or is about to begin. These fertility treatments may include: fertility drugs, IUI, ICI and surgery. In the case of surgery, they may see you for the first and second appointment just before the surgery and once more after the surgery. In the other cases you could see your client for two sessions during their treatment and another one after they have had their pregnancy test.

### An overview of The 3 Session Plan For ART

In session one, spend a short time on goal setting and focus on doing deep relaxation and *Mental Rehearsal*. In effect, combine Stage 1, 2 and 5 (*Outcome, Balance* and *Prepare*). In the following session, combine relaxation and visualisation (*Balance* and *Enhance*), using scripts and techniques that would be most useful for the client's current stage of medical treatment. If possible, do some *Resource Gathering* (*Balance*) to build ego strength and equip the client to deal with the results of treatment. Also, encourage them to come back when they have heard their results. If the treatment has been successful, you can work together to maintain pregnancy and *Prepare* for birth and parenthood. If the treatment has been unsuccessful, aim to provide *Support* in whatever way would be most useful for them.

Given the time constraints, and the fact that they are in the middle of medical treatment, it probably won't be possible to work through some of the client's deeper issues that need resolution, except in the rare case where the client requests this.

The Fertile Body Method

*The 3 Session Plan outline*

**Session 1**: Outcome, Balance and Prepare

Sending out a questionnaire may be a good way to save some time in the first session.
Because time is often limited in this session, (due to goal setting and case history taking) a distilled or shortened version of the suggested approaches can be used. Combine sections of the most appropriate scripts and techniques based on the medical treatment that your client is undergoing and their goal for therapy.

*Outcome*: set the goal for therapy and take the case history.

- Explain how hypnotherapy works, and how it may be helpful for them.

- The following questions may be useful in setting the goal:
  - What are your expectations for hypnotherapy?
  - In what way would you like this therapy to help you as you go through your medical treatment?
  - What would you like to change as a result of seeing me?
  - How will those changes be good for you?

- Typically, women who consult a hypnotherapist when they are about to start or have already started medical treatment want to feel calmer and more relaxed and/or to have a positive mental focus.

- Ask case history questions to determine the client's inner resources, positive past experiences, interests and how they like to relax. This information will be very helpful in choosing the most appropriate language, suggestions and approaches.

*Balance*: deep relaxation.

- There are a wide range of techniques that can induce deep relaxation, including:
  - *7:11 Breathing*
  - *Breathing Colour*
  - *Healing Green Light*
  - *Favourite Place.*

- Choose the approach that will be most effective for your client.

- Teach them how to induce relaxation for themselves. This can be taught as a form of *Self-Hypnosis*, or by teaching them one of the self-help tools that induce relaxation such as the *Mini-Break Anchor*.

*Prepare*: Mental Rehearsal.

- Using guided visualisation and suggestion, take your client through their fertility treatment so that they can see themselves thinking, feeling, behaving and responding to the treatment in the way that they would like to.

- If it is relevant for your client, future pace them to a situation in which they have anticipated some difficulty, so that they can mentally rehearse handling the situation in the way that they would like to.

- *Mental Rehearsal* can also be used to help the client see how they will benefit from using what they have learnt in the session with you.

*Self-help tools*

One or two of the following self-help tools can be taught to your client:

- *Mini-Break Anchor*: can be used to induce relaxation on the spot, which is particularly helpful for use before clinic appointments, during the time spent waiting for treatment, getting results, scans, and so on.

- *Orange Dots*: can be used to trigger and reinforce a positive visualisation used during the session.

- *Self-Hypnosis*: for daily relaxation and visualisation.

- *7:11 Breathing:* to induce a feeling of relaxation and calm.

**Session 2**: Balance and Enhance

*Balance*: deep relaxation.

*Enhance*: visualisations, metaphor and other techniques.

- The following scripts and techniques may be useful for enhancing the effectiveness of medical treatment:
    - *Conception:* for IUI, ICI, donation and surrogacy.
    - *Embryo Transfer:* for egg, sperm or embryo donation.

- *Implantation*: to visualise the fertilised egg implanting.
- *Visualisation:* for anaesthetics and fertility drugs working effectively (for use with fertility drugs such as Clomid).
- *Primal Image*: to prepare the womb to receive the fertilised embryo for IUI, ICI and donation. The Primal Image can also be used for surgical procedures. In step 2 of this process you would ask 'And how will that image change when this surgery has been successful?'
- *Control Room.*
- *Apposition Of Opposites.*
- *Fertility Garden.*
- *Inner Guide.*

- All these scripts and techniques are suggestions and should be tailored and adapted to suit your client's situation. The script or technique you choose to use will largely be influenced by the current stage of their fertility treatment.

- Incorporate suggestions for the client to repeat the visualisation which you have done together daily during *Self-Hypnosis*.

- You could also record the hypnosis session so that your client can take it home and listen to it each day.

**Session 3**: Prepare and Support

*For women who have become pregnant*
Women who become pregnant as a result of fertility treatment may have mixed reactions to the news. Some may feel relieved, excited and pleased while others may be filled with fear and anxiety. They may be anxious about the possibility of miscarriage, being pregnant, giving birth or becoming parents. For those clients who have just had surgery, this session can help support their recovery as well as prepare them for conception.

*Balance*: deep relaxation.

*Prepare*: visualisation.

- The following techniques may be appropriate for maintaining the pregnancy and preparing for parenthood:
  - *Inner Guide*
  - *Fertility Garden*
  - *Three Steps Forward*: to reduce anxiety about pregnancy.

- *Primal Image*: to maintain the pregnancy to full term for women who have previously miscarried or are anxious about miscarriage. In step 2 of this process you would ask 'How will that image change when you know that your body can carry this baby to full term?'
- *Pseudo-orientation / Future Pacing*: to pregnancy and/or birth.
- *Self-Integration Dissociation*: to release any anxiety or fear and to develop inner resources that may be needed during this time.

• To support pregnancy:
- *Visualisation*: mentally rehearsing a positive pregnancy.

• For those who have had surgery the following techniques may help to enhance their fertility and prepare them for pregnancy:
- *Primal Image*: this can help their unconscious mind register the positive changes that have resulted from the surgery.
- *Apposition Of Opposites*: to bring all the systems of their body into balance after the surgery, or to balance the systems of the body to create a optimal fertile state.
- *Pseudo-orientation / Future Pacing* to see the positive effects of the surgery and the beneficial changes that happen as a result.
- Direct suggestion: for the body to recovery well from surgery.

*Self-help tools*

• *Affirmations*: these are particularly good for women who are anxious about the pregnancy not going to term. For example: I trust in my body's ability to hold and support a healthy growing baby.

• Daily exercise: for example, suggest that your client rubs their belly every day to reinforce their confidence in their capacity to maintain the pregnancy.

*For women whose fertility treatment has not resulted in pregnancy*

*Balance*: deep relaxation, challenge beliefs and self-care.

• Relaxation can be very therapeutic for women whose medical treatment has been unsuccessful. Relaxation suggestions are focused on 'recharging, renewing and re-energising' rather than relaxation suggestions which may promote lethargy and depression such as 'heaviness and tiredness'.

- Restore and maintain balances when treatment has failed by addressing any unhealthy beliefs which the client may have about the treatment's failure, such as 'I am a failure' or 'I don't deserve to have a baby'. The following techniques may be helpful:
    - *Cognitive Restructuring*
    - *DoorsOfPerception*
    - *PartsWork*
    - *Self-Integration Dissociation.*

- Ask questions and discuss ways in which your client can take care of herself at this time as it will help improve her wellbeing and lift her mood. Examples of the questions I may ask include:
    - *If you were really loving yourself at this time, what would you be doing? What would you be thinking?*
    - *What do you know you need right now?*
    - *If you could do anything at this time, what would you do? In what way do you know that would be good for you? What other ways do you know of doing that?*

- Build and develop inner resources to help the client cope more easily with their disappointment and loss. This can be done using direct suggestion or resource gathering techniques.

*Support*: acknowledge the loss.

- Allow them time to talk about how they feel.

- Recommend that they give themselves some time and space to grieve. Perhaps suggest the *Grief Ceremony* for homework.

- Encourage them to talk openly with their partner.

- Discuss what their future options are and provide support for their decision making.

- Often treatments using stimulation drugs or IUI are done for a few months before couples are faced with a decision about what to do next. If the early cycles have not worked then help the client recognise that the next cycle may work. Some techniques that are useful for renewing hope are:
    - *Fertility Garden*
    - *Inner Guide*
    - *Out of The Box*

- *Healing White Light*
- *Pseudo-orientation / Future Pacing.*

*Self-help tools*

- *Nurturing*

- *Cognitive Restructuring*: to challenge any unhealthy beliefs which may arise as a result of the treatment not succeeding

- *Self-Talk SUDS*: to reduce negative self-talk

- *Emotional Bank Account*: for self-care

- *Grief Ceremony*: to acknowledge and process the loss

- *Self-Hypnosis*: to access and connect with their inner resources.

> *Case study: The 3 Session Plan For ART*
> *An example of how the 3 Session Plan for ART can be used and adapted.*
>
> A young Indian woman travelled from abroad to see me. She had been diagnosed with anovulation and as a result had been given fertility drugs to help stimulate ovulation. She had been taking these drugs for six months without conceiving. She only had a couple of weeks in London so we booked three appointments quite close together. When she came to see me for her first appointment, she had just started a new menstrual cycle. She was particularly concerned about the negative effects of the fertility drugs and explained to me that she didn't like taking medication of any kind. She had become increasingly anxious about her failure to conceive and felt that her fertility problems had completely knocked her self-confidence. She told me that in her culture an inability to conceive was shameful, and women without children were pitied. She felt under enormous pressure to have a child, and believed that her worth depended on it.
>
> In our first session together we spent quite a lot of time creating the goal. She found the process very empowering and said that it made her realise that there were many things that she did have control over and could change. Her goal for therapy included the following:
>
> - To realise her worth irrespective of whether she has children or not.
>
> - To reduce her stress levels so that she can feel more calm and relaxed.
>
> - To support her body and help enhance the effectiveness of the medication she was taking.
>
> - To discover some of her life goals and the different ways that she could have a meaningful life.
>
> Guided by her goal, our sessions focused on *Stage 2: Balance*: emotional, mental and physical. In the first session I taught her how to achieve deep relaxation using hypnosis. We spent some time in each session refining this tool so that she could use it every day to increase relaxation and reinforce our work together. After our first session I gave her the homework task of challenging the belief that her 'worth depends on whether she has children or not'.

In our second session I used the *Doors Of Perception* to help develop her new belief: 'I am a worthwhile woman irrespective of whether I have children or not.'

During the trance session she had a very powerful experience. As she walked through the door where she believed and knew that she was 'worthwhile irrespective of whether she had children or not' she saw her life unfolding before her. She described how she became aware that even if she did not have children she could live a very happy and fulfilled life. She saw her future helping other women in her country who were experiencing some of the difficulties she had been through. In the trance state she realised that the experience she'd been through and all the heartache she'd endured had provided her with everything she needed for being able to help others. I asked her to tell me more about the qualities that she had which would allow her to do this kind of work. When she had identified all the ways in which she was equipped to help others, she told me that she felt a huge weight lifting from her chest and shoulders.

I suggested that she take some time when she got home to make a collage that captured the essence of what she had seen as her life goal as well as the skills, tools, experiences and gifts that made it possible for her to fulfil it.

In our final session we used the *Healing White Light* to help enhance the effectiveness of her medication and release any excess medication so that her body could remain in a state of wellbeing. I chose this technique for her because she had an interest in prana healing and had previously described her experience of 'the healing force' as being a white light. I suggested that she repeat this visualisation during her *Self-Hypnosis* sessions at home.

At the end of the session I asked her to access her new belief, 'I am a worthwhile woman irrespective of whether I have children or not.' As she was silently and mentally saying the words to herself, I suggested that she recall the vision she had of herself fulfilling her life goal. I asked her to become aware of the positive feelings that arose as she did this and asked her to locate them in her body, and describe them as a colour, shape, temperature and texture. At the end of her final session I suggested that she repeat this *Affirmation* on her own every day as a way to reinforce this belief. This self-help tool was taught to her in the last session as a way to help her *Maintain* the changes.

## *The* Fertile Body Method *and IVF*

*How hypnosis and mind-body approaches can help people going through IVF*

- Clients can be taught how to achieve a deep state of relaxation using hypnosis that will help reduce their stress levels significantly and increase calmness throughout the IVF cycle.

- Hypnotherapy can be used to equip them with tools and inner resources that will help them cope better and handle an unsuccessful outcome more easily.

- Hypnosis can be used to help them prepare mentally, emotionally and physically for IVF. This preparation can range from making positive lifestyle changes, to changing limiting beliefs, to eliminating a needle phobia.

- Hypnosis can help enhance the treatment and increase the chances of a successful IVF outcome.

- Hypnosis can help reduce anxiety about miscarriage and support women who conceive to maintain pregnancy to full term.

- At times when difficult decisions and choices need to be made during or after IVF, hypnotherapy can support couples to make decisions more easily.

*The stages of an IVF cycle*

There are six distinct phases in IVF treatment. It can vary slightly from clinic to clinic, but the typical pattern of treatment is as follows:

- IVF preparation
  This phase of treatment includes all the necessary tests and scans that assess the suitability of the couple. Depending on the couple's diagnosis, test results and previous IVF response, a treatment protocol will be selected.
    - Couples on the long protocol take medication in the form of a nasal spray or injection that shuts down the normal hormonal response. This is known as down regulation and lasts about 10 to14 days.

- Those on the short protocol do not require this down regulation phase. They start ovarian stimulation treatment at the beginning of their menstrual cycle. This protocol is usually recommended for older women, women with high FSH, or those who have not responded well to stimulation during a previous cycle.
- A flare-up cycle is often used for women over 38 who have reduced ovarian reserve. This involves a few days of down regulation followed by the stimulation phase.

- Ovarian stimulation (10 to 14 days)
  The ovaries are stimulated to produce eggs with daily fertility drug injections. There is regular monitoring of the development of the eggs and uterine lining. These injections are typically done at home and the couple is responsible for administering the injections themselves.

- Egg collection and sperm collection
  When the eggs have developed sufficiently they are extracted under anaesthesia or sedation. Generally this surgical procedure is quite straightforward, but sometimes it can be uncomfortable and some women may experience some bruising after the surgery. On the day of egg collection the man is required to provide a sample of sperm which is then combined with the eggs. Cell division in the fertilised embryos is monitored in the lab. Two days after egg collection, progesterone is administered to help prepare the lining of the womb for pregnancy.

- Embryo transfer (ET)
  The transfer of the embryos back into the womb can happen anywhere between two and five days after collection, depending on the way the embryos mature. This procedure is usually pain free and done without the use of sedation. The woman is required to have a full bladder so that the womb can be seen more easily. A small catheter is passed through the cervix and a maximum of two embryos are transferred back into the uterus for implantation. The unused embryos can be frozen and used at a later time. Often two days of bed rest is recommended after the ET.

- The two week wait
  This phase is a time of waiting to find out whether or not the treatment has been successful and implantation has occurred.

- Results
  After two weeks it is sometimes recommended that the woman go into the clinic to have a pregnancy test done. Alternatively the results of the test are given by phone.

## The 4 Session Plan For IVF

This treatment plan is designed to enhance the effectiveness of each phase of IVF using four sessions of hypnotherapy.

*The 4 Session Plan* can begin any time before IVF is due to start. The next three sessions are best scheduled:

- During stimulation

- Before implantation

- During the two week wait. (Depending on your client, it may be more beneficial to have the final session after the results.)

To avoid any unnecessary emotional disturbance, I would not recommend doing any *Stage 3: Resolve* work in the middle of an IVF cycle. During the IVF treatment, hypnotherapy is best used as a tool to enhance the effectiveness of the drugs, build inner resources and increase relaxation and calmness.

For maximum benefit, this protocol should include all four sessions, but it can be tailored to suit your client's schedule and finances. It may be useful to send out a questionnaire before therapy begins so that time in the session can be used efficiently.

*The 4 Session Plan* outlined below includes techniques, scripts, self-help tools and homework. It is particularly suitable for women who have limited time and money and would like to use hypnotherapy during IVF. This plan is designed to:

- *Balance*: reduce stress and anxiety and increase relaxation

- *Balance*: create a healthy mental attitude

- *Balance*: develop inner resources to be able to cope

- *Prepare*: for IVF treatment physically, mentally and emotionally

- *Prepare*: the womb to receive a fertilised embryo

- *Enhance*: the effectiveness of medication

- *Enhance*: the chances of a successful outcome

- *Support*: after the IVF treatment has been completed.

## The 4 Session Plan For IVF

**Session 1**: Outcome, Balance and Prepare

*Timing*
This session is designed for before IVF treatment begins.

*Session aims*

- To inform the client about hypnosis and the ways it can be used
- To set the goal for therapy
- To reduce stress and anxiety and increase relaxation
- To create a healthy mental attitude and build inner resources
- To prepare for IVF.

*Considerations*
To help the client prepare for the IVF treatment you may need to ask them 'How will you know you are mentally, emotionally and physically prepared for your IVF treatment?' The answer to this question will determine the emphasis of this session. So, for example, a client who says they will know because they will feel okay about injecting themselves will need to use this session to reduce anxiety about needles. Someone who says that they will know because they will be feeling physically well may need to address balance and lifestyle, and so on.

Creating a healthy mental attitude might require the therapist to explain a little bit about what such a mental attitude is – acknowledging the possibility that the treatment may not work, but giving all their thoughts and attention to the possibility that it could work. Using visualisations and other techniques to focus on the desired outcome can have a positive effect on the way a client's body responds to the drugs and also helps to reduce worry and negative thinking.

Clients who have had repeated IVF failures are likely to be thinking and believing that the next cycle won't work. Generally people do recognise how going into the IVF treatment with this attitude isn't helpful. The case study below describes how I worked with someone who was feeling this way. It is important in cases such as these to build up inner resources so that the client knows they can cope with an unsuccessful outcome.

*Treatment*
In some ways the first session of this plan is the most tailored because the aim is to help the client feel prepared for their treatment. Since feeling prepared will mean different things to different people, the techniques you choose can vary widely. These techniques and scripts are generally very helpful in establishing balance and preparing for IVF:

- *Breathing Colour*: to reduce stress.

- *Creating A Fertile Body*.

- *Connect With The Inner Body*: to restore balance to the reproductive system.

- *Apposition Of Opposites*: to balance the systems of the body so that they're in an optimal state for medical treatment.

- *Self-Integration Dissociation*: to build inner resources, to feel ready and prepared for treatment and to have a healthy mental attitude towards IVF treatment.

- *Control Room*: to set control to optimum levels for IVF treatment.

- *Inner Guide*: for guidance about what changes to make in preparation for IVF or to receive support and resources from the adviser.

- *Resource Gathering*: to access useful inner resource such as strength, confidence or calmness.

- *IVF Preparation:* to create a positive expectation.

- *Pseudo-orientation / Future Pacing*: to see the whole IVF cycle happening as they would like it to happen.

*Homework and self-help tools*

- *Self-Hypnosis*: for relaxation and to practise any visualisations done in the session to help prepare the mind and body for treatment.

- *Nurturing*: to increase feelings of calmness and wellbeing.

- *Cognitive Restructuring*: to shift any limiting or unhealthy beliefs that may be creating anxiety.

- *Creative Task*: to create a piece of art that represents the way they would like to be thinking, feeling and behaving through the IVF treatment or a collage of all the resources they have that will help them through the treatment.

- *Affirmation*: to invoke a healthy mental and emotional state for the IVF treatment, for example, 'I can be calm and relaxed throughout my IVF procedure knowing that I can deal with whatever happens'.

**Session 2:** Balance, Enhance and Prepare

*Timing*
This session is designed for the stimulation phase of IVF.

*Session aims*

- To manage the administration of the drugs

- To increase the effectiveness of the drugs and respond well to the treatment

- To decrease the negative side effects of the drugs and create emotional stability

- To produce healthy, viable eggs

- To prepare for egg collection.

*Considerations*
Administering the drugs can be quite a complicated and demanding daily chore and many people find it very stressful. The stimulation stage of the cycle is particularly important because if few or no eggs are produced, the cycle will have to be abandoned.

The daily practice of having to inject stimulation drugs can be used as an opportunity for positive visualisation, focused intention and treating this daily task as a sacred ritual. If it is appropriate for your client, you could suggest that she and her partner do the injections together so that they can both be engaged in the process. You could suggest to your client that she thinks of ways in which she could make the daily injections a special ritual rather than a chore. Some of my clients have taken this on board and found that it has made a profound difference to their IVF experience.

A woman who was going through her third IVF treatment decided to create a special place in her house that she dedicated to her unborn child. She built a beautiful altar which had pictures of children and a pregnant woman, a congratulations card, a small pot of earth with a sprouting seed, fresh fruit, candles and her injection paraphernalia. When it was time to inject herself, she would sit in front of the altar for a few minutes, breathing deeply and focusing her mind on her intention to have a baby. When she felt relaxed and focused she would prepare the injection and as she administered it she would think about it bringing her one step closer towards her baby. She told me that by making it into a sacred ritual she had begun to look forward to it rather than dread it as she had done in the past. She experienced far fewer side effects and produced more eggs than she had in previous cycles.

Another woman chose to do her injections with her husband. They set aside half an hour for their ritual and used it as an opportunity to slow down and just be together. They would lay a red blanket down on the floor, light a few candles and put some soothing music on. Her husband would prepare the injection and then they would lie together on the blanket, relaxing and enjoying the physical contact. When they both felt calm and ready she would close her eyes and he would administer the injection. As he was injecting the medication she would visualise it as a golden liquid flowing to the parts of her body that needed it. She would see her ovaries responding well to this liquid and then imagine all the excess liquid being released and cleared away. We had done this visualisation together in our session and she found it really helpful to do as part of her ritual.

*Treatment*

The following scripts and techniques are recommended and should all be combined with deep relaxation and inner resource building:

- *IVF Preparation*: visualisation of a golden liquid to enhance egg production, visualisation to thicken the womb lining and prepare for egg collection.

- *Healing White Light*: with suggestions for supporting the effectiveness of the drugs and the light cleansing and clearing any excess medication.

- *Primal Image*: for the ovaries and/or reproductive system. Making changes to the image if they need so that they know their ovaries/system is responding well.

- *Apposition Of Opposites*: to balance the systems of the body so that the medication can be effective.

- *Body Talk*: can be used and adapted if your client is experiencing any negative side effects that they would wish to minimise. It can also be adapted to allow your client to talk to different parts of their body to find out what is needed to help increase the effectiveness of the drugs.

- *Control Room*: to make adjustments to the controls to ensure their body can respond well without any unnecessary side effects.

*Homework and self-help tools*

- Injection ritual.

- *Quick Body Scan*: to maintain body awareness and recognise needs, as well as to maintain physical relaxation.

- *Nurturing*: self-care is very important at this time. Remind your client to drink plenty of water to flush away toxins from the medication and to rest as much as possible.

- *Self-Hypnosis*: doing the *Apposition Of Opposites* to maintain balance in the mind, heart and body.

- *Self-Hypnosis*: visit the *Control Room* to maintain body's appropriate and healthy response to drugs.

- *Self-Hypnosis*: to repeat positive visualisations of good egg production and a good egg collection.

- *Self-Hypnosis*: glove anaesthesia (for more information about glove anaesthesia please refer to Waxman, 1998) if there is any post-operative pain.

- *7:11 Breathing*: to reduce anxiety about the egg collection procedure.

**Session 3:** Balance, Enhance and Prepare

*Timing*
This session is designed for before Embryo Transfer.

*Session aims*

- To prepare the womb to receive the embryos.

- To increase the chances of implantation.

- To increase blood flow to the uterus.

*Considerations*
The research study that showed that hypnosis could double the success of embryo transfer (Levitas, 2006) used deep relaxation and suggestions for welcoming the embryos into the womb. The hypnosis was carried out while the patients were undergoing embryo transfer. One of the possible explanations for the increased success is due to the relaxation of the uterine muscles, making implantation easier.

I mention this study because it indicates that actually being in a state of deep hypnotic relaxation during the transfer is beneficial. Teaching your client *Self-Hypnosis* means that they will be able to enter a relaxed state during the transfer. I also recommend that clients listen to the CD or MP3 that I have made for them during transfer. Some clients have said that it has been possible for them to do this while others have found that listening to a portable CD player or iPod has not been possible or allowed at their clinic.

*Treatment*
The following scripts and techniques are recommended:

- *Embryo Transfer*

- *Fertility Garden*

- *Inner Guide:* to help prepare the womb and create the right conditions for implantation to occur

- *Conception*: visualisation to see the fertilised embryo growing and implanting

- *Primal Image:* to create a womb that is welcoming, nurturing, safe and loving.

*Homework and self-help tools*

- *Self-Hypnosis:* visualisation for implantation and blood flow to the uterus.

- *Self-Hypnosis:* for relaxation of the uterine muscles during embryo transfer.

- *Creative Tasks:* create a collage showing the womb as a welcoming, nurturing, safe and loving environment.

**Session 4:** Balance, Enhance and Support

*Timing*
This session is designed for the two week wait.

*Session aims*

- To increase levels of calmness and relaxation during this time

- Encourage rest and stillness

- Create a healthy focus

- Build inner resources to be able to cope with the outcome of IVF.

*Considerations*

The two week wait can be a challenging and anxious time for many women. Women should be encouraged to have a couple of days' bed rest after the transfer and to maintain a low level of activity during the two weeks.

Because this is a time of rest and doing less, many women find it incredibly hard to maintain a positive mind-set. Often the time is spent feeling anxious and worrying about whether the treatment will work or not. The *Worry Less* tool in *Stage 2: Balance* (Page 78) can be very useful at this time. I also suggest to clients that they think about useful and enjoyable ways of spending this restful time. In response to this suggestion, one client used the time to write a short children's story, and another printed out her holiday photographs and made a beautiful scrapbook with them. *Creative Tasks* and positive visualisation are an effective way to maintain a healthy focus of attention.

Therapists often ask me whether it is beneficial and appropriate during the two week wait to do visualisations of the pregnancy and holding the baby. I'm not really sure that there is a conclusive answer to this question. I believe that visualising the desired outcome can be beneficial but for some people it may provoke anxiety. I also recognise that in some cases it may be 'setting them up' for disappointment. At this stage of treatment I would suggest letting the client lead. General pseudo-orientation with permissive suggestions will allow the client to choose to visualise whatever is most appropriate for them.

*Treatment*

The following scripts and techniques are recommended:

- *Conception*: to visualise the egg fertilising and developing.

- *Healing Green Light*: for deep relaxation.

- *Self-Integration Dissociation*: to release worry and build inner resources.

- *Resource Gathering*: to feel strong enough to cope with the outcome.

- *Inner Guide:* to ask for advice on how best to support the growing embryo during this time.

- Time distortion suggestions: to create a perception of the two weeks just flying by.

- *Pseudo-orientation / Future Pacing*: to see the embryo developing and growing.

- Direct suggestion: for calmness, rest and a positive mental focus.

*Homework and self-help tools*

- *Creative Tasks*: to give the mind a positive focus during this time.

- *Orange Dots*: as a cue to trigger a positive visualisation. For example: 'And whenever you see that orange dot on your watch face, you will see your baby being safely held and nourished in your womb.'

- *Gratitudes*: to increase feelings of wellbeing and maintain a healthy perspective.

- *Mini-Break Anchor*: to create calmness and clarity when receiving the results.

- *Meditation*: to cultivate calmness.

- *Cognitive Restructuring*: to challenge any unhealthy beliefs that may arise as a result of unsuccessful treatment.

- *Worry Less*: to maintain a positive focus.

## Case study: repeated IVF failure and negative expectation

A few days before Dina's fifth IVF cycle was due to begin, she came to see me for the first time. I asked her how she would know the four sessions we planned to have together had been helpful. She said that if she was able to believe that it is possible for this IVF cycle to work, she would know it had helped. I asked her how she thought believing this would be good for her and she quickly answered that there was no point going into the treatment believing it was going to fail. At saying that, she laughed and said that if she really did believe it was going to fail, why would she be bothering to put herself through the whole ordeal in the first place?

I asked why else she thought believing the treatment would fail was pointless. After some thought, Dina said that if her body was receiving messages from her mind about not being pregnant while she was pumping all sorts of drugs into her system that were telling her body to be pregnant, the confusion was likely to result in stress and failure.

Although she knew that thinking like this was not helpful, she did not know how to stop herself from thinking this way. As part of the goal setting, I asked her to tell me how she would prefer to be thinking, feeling and behaving as she went through the IVF cycle. This information provided us both with a very full picture of what the change would be like for her.

In our first session together I used the *Healing White Light* to instil deep relaxation and calmness. I gave suggestions that the light could help her clear and cleanse any negative emotional residue from her past IVF experiences, so that her memories remained intact but the emotional content associated with those memories was cleared and washed away by the light.

I used *Parts Work* to help her access the part of herself that was responsible for believing the IVF cycle wouldn't work. The main purpose of using *Parts Work* here was to help her understand the positive intention of the part and to gather the resources she needed so that part no longer needed to dominate her experience.

Dina saw that the part responsible for believing IVF would fail was trying to protect her from more disappointment and sadness. I suggested that she thank that part for trying to protect her and explain to it that she really needed it to work for her in a more helpful way. She told the part that she needed to be able to believe the IVF could work. She asked the part if there was anything it needed in order to protect her without having to hold onto the belief that the treatment wouldn't work.

> Dina had imagined the part responsible for believing the IVF wouldn't work as a solid stone wall blocking her field of vision. When she asked it what it needed an image came to mind of an invisible force field. She identified this resource as inner strength and endurance. I asked her to offer this to the part responsible and as she did that, she saw the wall move from her field of vision to somewhere inside her. The invisible force field had replaced the stone wall, continuing to protect her and also allowing her to see and think more clearly. I asked her to describe how the part had changed and she said that it was now using its powers of protection as an inner strength rather than a barrier. I asked her to connect with the strength and endurance that was now within her. When she was feeling strong and safe, I asked her to look in front of her, through the invisible force protecting her, and to tell me what she was able to see ahead of her now.
>
> Tears began to flow down her cheeks as she described seeing herself pregnant. I reinforced our work together by reminding her that she could continue to be connected with her inner strength which would allow her to continue to be able to see the very real possibility that this treatment could work.
>
> This first session described above includes *Stage 1: Outcome* and *Stage 2: Balance*. The *Healing White Light* helped restore emotional balance and *Parts Work* helped to restore mental balance by building inner resources and ego strength.

For clients who are struggling with this kind of negative expectation, the following explanation may be helpful:

> *Having a negative expectation for the outcome of the treatment in an attempt to protect yourself from disappointment if the treatment fails is a faulty strategy. Firstly, the negative expectation produces a state of anxiety because of this anticipated result. Secondly, focusing your attention in this way sends mixed signals to your body about what your intention is. Thirdly, the negative expectation doesn't actually prevent the feelings you will have if the treatment does not work. This kind of strategy doesn't actually serve you in any way. Accepting that you will feel disappointed if it doesn't work, gives you the freedom to use your mental and emotional energy in a helpful and supportive way.*

## The Complete Plan For IVF

This plan combines the six stages of the *Fertile Body Method* and *The 4 Session Plan For IVF*. The complete plan can range from six to fifteen or more sessions and is for those who are seeking a thorough and in-depth approach to supporting and enhancing IVF.

The six stages of the *Fertile Body Method* take place before IVF treatment begins and aim to address and resolve any issues that may be affecting fertility and the successful outcome of treatment. It would be preferable to see the client a minimum of four weeks before IVF treatment begins, so that you can work through the relevant aspects of Stages 1 to 6 of the *Fertile Body Method* before beginning *The 4 Session Plan For IVF*. This will ensure that the client is in the best possible state for IVF treatment and that any relevant issues have been addressed.

The way in which you use the six stages of the *Fertile Body Method* will depend upon the client's goal for therapy, as well as their unique history and current situation. For more information about the six stages of treatment and how to construct your treatment plan, please refer to Section B (Page 23).

---

### Case study: reaching acceptance

Working thoroughly and deeply with someone in preparation for their IVF treatment can be very rewarding. In one particular case, I realised that following the *Complete Plan* really allowed my client to experience her fourth and last IVF cycle as an empowering experience. Although the IVF treatment did not result in pregnancy, the client felt really good throughout and was left feeling that she had overcome her fear of not being able to have children. Overcoming her fear allowed her to be able to move on with her life and look back on her fertility journey as a growing and healing experience.

During her hypnotherapy treatment we spent a lot of time focusing on various aspects of *Balance* in preparation for her IVF cycle. Through our work with IMRs, *Parts Work*, *Cognitive Restructuring* and *Resource Gathering* she began to recognise how the emotional pain that she was experiencing was as a direct result of her resisting the reality of her situation. Her frustration, anger, anxiety and fear were all a result of her refusal to accept the possibility of not having a child. Once she realised this, we could begin working towards finding acceptance.

In our fourth session together we reviewed her goal, and using the Solution Focused Therapy scale (Page 35), began to break her goal 'To find acceptance …' down into manageable steps so that she could first experience acceptance for small, easy things in her life and slowly work towards feeling acceptance for the possibility that she may not have her own children.

Acceptance is a concept that can easily be grasped intellectually, but learning to live in a state of acceptance can take time and practice. It is a continual process of learning to let go and surrender. She was concerned that if she did surrender to the possibility that she might not have children, she was somehow going to make that possibility a reality. Using *Apposition Of Opposites* she was able to find her own inner balance between acceptance and intention: accepting that she was having problems conceiving and that she may not have her own child while still having the intention of conceiving and becoming a mother.

In the following session, *Self-Integration Dissociation* was particularly useful for her as it helped her identify what inner resources she may need in order to be able to find acceptance. She recognised that she needed to be able to trust herself and the process of life in order to accept that things were okay the way they were and that everything she was experiencing was a necessary part of her life's journey.

As part of her homework I had given her the task of experimenting with how she could accept the loud disturbing noises that the builders next door had been making while she was trying to work. When we met again she told me that on one particular occasion when she recognised how frustrated she was feeling about the incessant noise, she had a very useful insight about acceptance: she asked herself what it was about this experience that was causing her to feel frustrated. She realised that it was because she was insisting that she had to have silence while she worked. She had decided that the noise was not supposed to be happening.

In that moment she decided to experiment with what it would be like if she decided that there was supposed to be noise and that it merely presented her with another way to experience working. As if by magic, her frustration dissolved and gave way to a feeling of relief. Her frustration had come from trying to work against the noise and she felt relieved to know that it was possible for her to work with the noise. She began to apply this to her fertility situation and was able to see how she could begin to acknowledge and accept it.

> By the time she started her IVF cycle she felt liberated from the fear and anxiety that had been overwhelming her for the past three years. Her body responded well to the medication and she felt energised and strong during each phase of the cycle. She used *Self-Hypnosis* to visualise the outcome she wanted and also practised how she could accept it if it did not work. She felt ready and prepared for anything.
>
> When she told me that the treatment had not worked, she was smiling and crying at the same time. She told me that for the first time in her life she had discovered what acceptance really meant. She had reached such a profound place of acceptance that she was filled with what she described as 'ecstasy'.
>
> Using *The Complete Plan For IVF* allowed her to have an empowering experience irrespective of the IVF results. It also meant that she felt ready to move on with the next chapter of her life because she felt at peace with how things had turned out. That's not to say that she didn't go through a time of grieving her loss, but rather that she was able to truly grieve because she had accepted her loss.

## *Adapting the IVF plan for egg, sperm and embryo donation*

The *4 Session Plan For IVF* can be adapted for couples who are using donated eggs, sperm or embryos.

It may be necessary to address some of the following issues in the first session:

- How does the woman feel about using donated sperm, eggs or embryos?
- How does her partner feel?
- What will they tell the child about how they were conceived?
- What are her concerns?

In cases of egg or embryo donation, the stimulation and egg collection stages of IVF will not be included. The woman will still need to take fertility drugs to prepare her body to receive the fertilised embryo; however, the second session of the plan can be adapted to focus on preparing her womb to receive the embryos. The following techniques may be useful:

- *Primal Image*: for the womb and reproductive system. Making changes to the image if they need to, so that they know that their system is responding well to the drugs and that their lining is thickening.

- *Apposition Of Opposites*: to balance the systems of the body so that the medication can be effective.

- *Control Room*: to make adjustments to the controls to ensure their body can respond well without any unnecessary side effects.

If the eggs or embryos are being donated, suggestions for bonding and connecting with them are beneficial as well as the *Conception* visualisation.

In cases where donated sperm is being used, the IVF process will be the same for the woman. You could use the *Primal Image* to help her access an image that represents one of the donated sperm. Then ask her what would need to change for her to feel that this sperm was the right one to fertilise her egg and become their baby. Making suggestions for bonding with the embryo before transfer can be a simple but direct way of overcoming any concerns about donated sperm, eggs and embryos.

## Section E: Resources

**Resources**
    Recommended reading .................................................................................351
    Useful websites ............................................................................................355
    Further study and support ...........................................................................359
    Glossary of terms ........................................................................................361
    Bibliography................................................................................................371
    Index ...........................................................................................................377
    Acknowledgements......................................................................................387

**Data CD**
A data CD, which contains various documents for the practitioner to download and print, including:
    Questionnaire – for men and woman
    Scripts and techniques – for therapists to customise and print
    Self-help tools – guide sheet handouts for clients
    Fertility Awareness Education Programme – handout for clients
    Finding meaning, purpose and direction – homework questions

## Recommended reading

*Fertility and Infertility*

HFEA (2008) *The HFEA guide to Infertility.* London.

Indichova, J. (1997) *Inconceivable: A Woman's Triumph Over Despair and Statistics.* New York: Broadway Books.

Lockwood, G., Anthony-Ackery, J., Meyers-Thompson, J. and Perkins, S. (2007) *Fertility and Infertility for Dummies.* Chichester: John Wiley and Sons.

Nicholas, M. (2006) *3 Steps to fertility.* London: Carroll and Brown Publishers Limited.

Singer, K. (2004) *The Garden of Fertility: A Guide to Charting Your Fertility Signals to Prevent or Achieve Pregnancy–Naturally–and to Gauge Your Reproductive Health.* New York: Avery.

*Mind-Body Medicine*

Dispenza, J. (2007) *Evolve your brain: the science behind changing your mind.* Deerfield Beach: Health Communications.

Lipton, D.B. (2005) *The Biology of Belief.* Santa Rosa: Mountain of Love/Elite Books.

Northrup, Christiane (1998) *Women's Bodies, Women's Wisdom: The Complete Guide to Women's Health and Wellbeing,* 2nd revised edition. London: Piatkus Books.

Pert, C.D. (1999) *Molecules of emotion: Why You Feel the Way You Feel.* New York: Touchstone.

Shapiro, D. (2008) *Your body speaks your mind.* London: Piakatus Books.

*Mind-Body / Hypnosis and Fertility*

Domar, A. (2002) *Conquering Infertility: Dr Alice Domar's guide to enhancing fertility and coping with infertility.* London: Viking Penguin.

Eastburn, L. (2006) *It's conceivable!* Victoria, Canada: Trafford Publishing.

Schwartz, J. (2008) *The mind-body fertility connection: The true pathway to conception.* Woodbury: Llewellyn Publications.

Lewis, R.P. (2004) *The Infertility Cure.* New York: Little, Brown and Company.

O'Neil, M.L. (2000) *Hypnofertility: The LeClair Method.* Pacific Palisades: Papyrus Press.

Payne, N.B. (1997) *The whole person fertility programme: A revolutionary mind-body process to help you conceive.* New York: Three Rivers Press.

*Menstrual Health*

Diamant, A. (2002) *The Red Tent.* London: Pan Books.

Northrup, Christiane (1998) *Women's Bodies, Women's Wisdom: The Complete Guide to Women's Health and Wellbeing,* 2nd revised edition. London: Piatkus Books.

Owen, L. (2008) *Her Blood is Gold.* Dorset: Archive Publishing.

Pope, A. (2001a) *Walking with the Genie: The Modern Woman's Menstrual Health Kit.* Self published.

Pope, A. (2001b) *The Wild Genie: the healing power of menstruation.* Bowral, Australia: Sally Milner Publishing.

Simpkins, C.A. and Simpkins, A.M. (2004) *Self Hypnosis For Women,* San Diego: Radiant Dolphin Press.

*Pregnancy and Childbirth*

Dick-Read, D.G. (2005) *Childbirth without Fear: The Principles and Practice of Natural Childbirth,* 4th edition. Pinter and Martin Ltd.

Gaskin, I.M. (1975) *Spiritual Midwifery.* Summertown, TN: Book Publishing Company.

Mongan, M. (2008) *HypnoBirthing: The Mongan Method: A natural approach to a safe, easier, more comfortable birthing,* 3rd edition. Dearfield Beach: Health Communications.

Motha, G. (2004) *The Gentle Birth Method: The Month-by-month Jeyarani Way Programme.* London: Thorsons.

Peterson, G. (1984) *Birthing Normally: A Personal Growth Approach to Childbirth.* Shadow and Light Publishing.

*Miscarriage, Abortion and Pregnancy Loss*

Kluger-Bell, K. (1998) *Unspeakable losses: Healing from Miscarriage, Abortion, and Other Pregnancy Losses.* New York: W.W. Norton.

Kübler-Ross, E. (2005) *On Grief and Grieving: Finding the Meaning of Grief Through the Five Stages of Loss.* Princeton: Scribner.

Nathanson Elkind, S. (1990) *Soul-Crisis: one woman's journey from abortion to renewal.* New York: Signet.

*Parenting*

Houser, P. M. (2007) *Fathers-To-Be Handbook: A Road Map for the Transition to Fatherhood.* Creative Life Systems.

Grille, R. (2008) *Heart to Heart Parenting.* ABC Books.

Grille, R. (2005) *Parenting For A Peaceful World.* Longueville Media.

*Hypnosis, Hypnotherapy and Psychotherapy*

De Shazer, S. (1985) *Keys to Solution in Brief Therapy.* New York: W.W. Norton.

De Shazer, S. (1994) *Words were Originally Magic.* New York: W.W. Norton.

Dilts, R., and DeLozier, J. (2000) *Encyclopedia of systemic NLP and NLP new coding.* Scotts Valley: NLP University Press.

Dryden, W. (2001) *Reason to Change: A Rational Emotive Behaviour Therapy (REBT) Workbook.* East Sussex: Brunner-Routledge.

Gilligan, S. (1997) *The Courage to Love: Principles and Practices of Self-relations Psychotherapy.* New York: W.W. Norton.

Hammond, D.C. (1990) *Handbook of hypnotic suggestions and metaphors.* New York: W.W. Norton.

O'Hanlon, B. and Beadle, S. (1999) *A guide to possibilty land.* New York: W.W. Norton.

Rossi, E.L. (2002) *The psychobiology of gene expression: Neuroscience and neurogenesis in hypnosis and the healing arts.* New York: W.W. Norton.

Rossi, E.L. and Cheek, D.B. (1994) *Mind-Body Therapy; ideodynamic healing in hypnosis.* New York: W.W. Norton.

Waxman, D. (1998) *Medical and Dental Hypnosis.* Bath: Bookcraft.

Wolinsky, S. (1991) *Trances People Live: Healing approaches in quantum psychology.* Las Vegas: The Bramble Company.

*Human Givens Approach*

Griffin, J. and Tyrrell, I. (2004) *How to lift depression fast.* Chalvington: HG Publishing.

Griffin, J. and Tyrrell, I. (2007) *How to master anxiety.* Chalvington: HG Publishing.

Griffin, J. and Tyrrell, I. (2004) *Human Givens: A new approach to emotional health and clear thinking.* Chalvington: HG Publishing.

## Useful Websites

**Adoption information line**
The most popular adoption internet site in the UK, providing the most relevant information on adoption.
www.adoption.org.uk

**BFS – British Fertility Society**
The British Fertility Society is a national multidisciplinary organisation representing professionals practising in the field of reproductive medicine.
www.britishfertilitysociety.org.uk

**BICA – British Infertility Counselling Association**
BICA is the only professional association for infertility counsellors and counselling in the UK.
www.bica.net

**BSCH – British Society of Clinical Hypnosis**
The BSCH is a national professional body whose aim is to promote and assure high standards in the practice of hypnotherapy. Registration demands good quality training, ethical practice and adherence to a code of conduct. A list of qualified hypnotherapists is available on the BSCH website.
www.bsch.org.uk

**COTS – Childlessness overcome through surrogacy**
Providing help and support to intended surrogate parents.
www.surrogacy.org.uk

**Daisy Network Premature Menopause Support Group**
The Daisy Network is a registered charity for women who have experienced a premature menopause.
www.daisynetwork.org.uk

**EFT – Emotional Freedom Techniques world centre**
EFT is an emotional, needle-free version of acupuncture based on the connection between the body's subtle energies, the emotions, and health.
www.emofree.com

**EMDR institute – Eye Movement Desensitisation and Reprocessing**
The EMDR institute provides information and links about the EMDR worldwide.
www.emdr.com

### Fathers-To-Be
Fathers-To-Be is an initiative to support men's understanding of pregnancy, birth and early fathering and supports expectant and new dads by reinforcing their relationship with themselves, their partners, their babies, and the health professionals caring for the family.
www.fatherstobe.org

### Foresight
Foresight is the **Association for the Promotion of Preconceptual Care,** which focuses on improving nutrition through diet and supplementation of vitamins and minerals, and combating substances which are poisonous to the body and to the environment.
www.foresight-preconception.org.uk

### Fostering information line
They provide comprehensive information on the fostering of children and foster care.
www.fostering.org.uk

### GHR – General Hypnotherapy Register
The GHR is a Professional Register of Hypnotherapists in the UK and is an administrating agency for both The General Hypnotherapy Standards Council and The Central Register of Stop Smoking Therapists.
www.general-hypnotherapy-register.com

### HFEA – The Human Fertilisation and Embryology Authority
The HFEA is the UK's independent regulator overseeing the use of gametes and embryos in fertility treatment and research.
www.hfea.gov.uk

### HGI – The Human Givens institute
The HGI provides information to the general public (via its website) about common areas of emotional distress and the best ways to treat them. It also includes information about the Human Givens Approach to emotional health and psychology including new insights into areas such as the causes of depression, the online register of accredited Human Givens therapists in private practice and a wealth of articles and case histories.
www.hgi.org.uk

### HypnoBirthing®
A complete antenatal education programme offering training to hypnotherapists, midwives and those who are interested in teaching couples how to use hypnosis for a safe and gentle birth experience.
www.hypnobirthing.co.uk/

**Infertility Network UK**
Infertility Network UK is the UK's leading infertility support network, offering information and support to anyone affected by fertility problems.
www.infertilitynetworkuk.com

**IPOFA – International Premature Ovarian Failure Association**
Offering information, help and support to women worldwide with premature ovarian failure.
www.pofsupport.org

**LCCH – London College of Clinical Hypnosis**
The LCCH was created in 1984 and provides training in hypnosis and hypnotherapy with the disciplines, skills and tuition necessary to practise hypnosis both soundly and ethically. The LCCH is in a collaborative partnership with Thames Valley University offering a recognised postgraduate programme in Clinical Hypnotherapy which can lead to a full Master's degree.
www.lcch.co.uk

**LCCH – Malaysia**
The LCCH Malaysia offers hypnotherapy training courses which are recognised internationally and at university level.
www.hypnosis-malaysia.com

**LCCH – Singapore**
The LCCH Singapore offers hypnotherapy training courses to professional and trainee healthcare workers in Singapore.
www.hypnosis-singapore.com

**META charity – Mind Education through Awareness**
META is a young and dynamic charity dedicated to making psychological health accessible to every child, parent and adult.
www.metacharity.org.uk

**MindFields College**
MindFields College offers training in a broad range of therapeutic skills and the most effective ways to treat a wide range of emotional distress (such as depression, anxiety, anger management, trauma, phobias, etc.) and work effectively with a variety of conditions. It also teaches a range of qualifications in Human Givens psychotherapy.
www.mindfields.org.uk

**Miscarriage Association**
The miscarriage association provides support and information for those suffering from the effects of pregnancy loss.
www.miscarriageassociation.org.uk

**NCT – the National Childbirth Trust**
The NCT help over a million mums and dads each year through pregnancy, birth and early days of parenthood by providing antenatal and post-natal courses, local support and reliable information.
www.nctpregnancyandbabycare.com

**Nourish**
Nourish has researched and developed a Conception Conditioning Programme which provides a convenient way to ensure that couples have the essential levels of nutrients, together with a healthy hormonal and digestive system, which are vital for conception and maintaining a healthy pregnancy. Nourish also run a satellite clinic network consisting of practitioners throughout the UK who offer specialist services in the area of pre-conceptual care.
www.nourish-fertility.com

**Sands – UK's stillbirth and neonatal death society**
Sands is an organisation which offers support to parents when their baby dies during pregnancy or after birth.
www.uk-sands.org

**School of Movement Medicine**
The school of movement medicine offers workshops and courses to help people discover and experience movement, meditation and ecstatic dance as a practice for transformation, artistic expression, wellness, personal growth and healing.
www.schoolofmovementmedicine.com

**The *Fertile Body Method* Therapist register**
For an up-to-date list of fully qualified *Fertile Body* therapists please visit the online register.
www.fertilebodytherapist.com

**The HALE Fertility Clinic**
The HALE Fertility Clinic in London offers men and woman with fertility problems a comprehensive mind-body approach to help support and enhance their fertility.
www.haleclinic.com

### The Wild Genie
The Wild Genie website has articles, books, links, workshops and information about restoring the integrity of the menstrual cycle, including transitions of menarche, pregnancy and childbirth and menopause.
www.wildgenie.com

## Further study and support

### The Fertile Body Website
The Fertile Body Website is a useful resource for therapists and members of the public. The site contains interesting articles about fertility and mind-body medicine, a selection of scripts, MP3 downloads and access to other useful websites, books, practitioners and more.
www.thefertilebody.com

### Webinars
A webinar is a 'live' hour-long interactive online seminar. Webinars are held throughout the year, each one covering a specific topic relating to the *Fertile Body Method*. Topics include: miscarriage, termination, natural conception, affects of stress on fertility, working with physical symptoms, menstrual health etc. If you would like to be on the mailing list to be notified of upcoming webinars, please email info@thefertilebody.com.

### Clinical Supervision
Sjanie is available for clinical supervision in person (London), by telephone or via Skype. These sessions can help to support you while working with fertility clients and are also a means to continue developing your knowledge and skills in this field. If you are planning a talk or a workshop about hypnosis and fertility, a supervision session can be used to get help structuring and preparing it. To arrange a clinical supervision session, please email info@thefertilebody.com.

## Glossary of terms
(Schwartz 2008; Fertility UK Glossary, 2009; Infertility Glossary, 2009)

| | |
|---|---|
| Abortion | The spontaneous or induced termination of pregnancy. |
| ACU | Assisted conception unit. |
| Amenorrhoea | The lack of menstruation. |
| Androgens | Male sex hormones. Most androgens are produced in the testes. Small amounts of androgens are also produced in a woman's ovaries and adrenal glands. |
| Anovulation | The absence of ovulation because an egg is not released from the ovary during the cycle. |
| Artificial insemination | The insertion of seminal fluid into the vagina, cervix or uterus by means other than sexual intercourse. The sperm may be from the husband or a donor. |
| Assisted conception | Any procedure where doctors assist with the conception process itself. |
| Assisted Reproductive Technology (ART) | Medical procedures carried out to facilitate the reproductive process, such as IVF, IUI, ICSI. |
| Autonomic Nervous System (ANS) | The part of the nervous systems that controls and regulates the automatic functions of the body, such as digestions, hormone production and heart rate. |
| Basal body temperature (BBT) | The temperature of the body at rest, taken immediately on waking, before any activity. |
| Blastocyst | An embryo that has developed for five to six days after fertilisation. |

| | |
|---|---|
| Cervical mucus | The secretion from the cells lining the cervix, which changes under the influence of the female sex hormones. The term 'cervical secretion' can be used synonymously. |
| Cervix | The lower portion of the uterus that projects into the vagina. |
| Conceive | To become pregnant. |
| Conception | Fusion of the sperm and the egg cell. |
| Contraception | The prevention of conception. |
| Contraceptive pill | Synthetic hormone/s taken orally to prevent pregnancy. |
| Corpus luteum (yellow body) | The endocrine gland, formed in the ruptured follicle after ovulation, which produces progesterone. If the egg is fertilised, the corpus luteum continues to produce hormones to support the early pregnancy. |
| Cortisol | A stress hormone produced by the adrenals which is known to inhibit the release of GnRH which stimulates ovulation. |
| Curettage/D and C | A surgical procedure used to scrape out the surface of the endometrium with an instrument called a curette. The procedure is often known as 'dilatation and curettage' or D and C, and is often done after a miscarriage. |
| Down regulation | The use of medication during fertility treatment which causes the ovaries to temporarily become inactive and prevents the release of eggs. |
| Dysmenorrhoea | Painful menstruation resulting from contractions in the uterus. |
| Dyspareunia | Painful or difficult intercourse. |

| | |
|---|---|
| Ectopic pregnancy | The implantation and development of a pregnancy outside of the uterus, usually in the Fallopian tube. |
| Egg | Gamete produced by a woman during her monthly cycle. Also called an Oocyte/Ovum. |
| Ejaculation | The release of seminal fluid from the penis during male orgasm. |
| Embryo | The initial stages of development of the unborn child from the fertilised egg, to around eight weeks after conception. |
| Endometriosis | The growth of endometrial tissue in areas other than the uterus, for example the Fallopian tubes or the ovaries. Endometriosis may contribute to fertility problems. |
| Endometrium | The inner lining of the uterus which is shed during menstruation. If conception occurs, the fertilised egg implants in the endometrium which provides nourishment for a developing embryo and foetus. |
| Fallopian tube | The tubes through which the ripened ovum is transported from an ovary towards the uterus. In the fertile phase sperm may pass from the uterus into the Fallopian tube where fertilisation normally takes place. |
| Fertile phase | The days of the menstrual cycle during which sexual intercourse may result in pregnancy. |
| Fertilisation | The fusion of a sperm with an ovum, normally in the outer end of the Fallopian tube, resulting in an embryo. |
| Fertility awareness | An essential basic education for understanding fertility throughout reproductive life. |

| | |
|---|---|
| Foetus | The term used for an unborn child from around eight weeks after conception (the time when all major organs are formed and it begins to resemble a human being) to the time of birth. |
| Fibroid | A benign fibrous and muscular growth of tissue in the muscular wall of the uterus. |
| Follicle | A small fluid-filled structure in the ovary which contains the ovum or egg cell. |
| Follicle stimulating hormone (FSH) | Hormone produced by the anterior pituitary gland that stimulates the ripening of follicles in the ovaries of females and the formation of sperm in the testes of males. FSH is available in synthetic form and can be used in fertility treatment. |
| Follicular phase | The pre-ovulatory phase characterised by the growth and development of the egg follicles. |
| Gamete intra-Fallopian transfer (GIFT) | Unfertilised egg and sperm placed into a woman's Fallopian tubes using a laparoscope. |
| Gonads | The primary sex glands – the testes in the male and the ovaries in the female. |
| Gonadotropin-releasing hormone (GnRH) | A hormone responsible for stimulating ovulation. |
| Hormone | A chemical substance which is produced and secreted by an endocrine gland. Hormones are carried by the blood to a target organ where they exert their effect. |
| HFEA | Human Fertilisation and Embryology Authority. A Government body which regulates clinics performing IVF and other treatments using sperm, eggs and embryos. |
| Hysterosalpingogram (HSG) | An X-ray of a dye test done to check for blockages in the Fallopian tubes. |

| | |
|---|---|
| Human chorionic gonadotrophin (HCG) | One of the main hormones unique to pregnancy. It is produced by the developing embryo from its earliest days. During IVF it is given to woman via injection to help mature the eggs. |
| Hypothalamus gland | A small gland located at the base of the brain which is considered to be the control centre for reproductive activity. |
| Hysterectomy | The surgical removal of the uterus. |
| Intracytoplasmic Sperm Injection (ICSI) | A single sperm is injected into a single egg in a laboratory. This technique is often used during IVF when there are problems with the sperm quality. |
| Idiopathic infertility | Infertility of unknown cause. |
| Implantation | The process by which the fertilised egg embeds in the endometrium. |
| Intra-uterine Insemination (IUI) | A fertility treatment during which a sample of sperm is inseminated into the uterus and conception occurs inside the body. |
| In vitro Fertilisation (IVF) | A method of assisted conception in which fertilisation takes place in a glass dish (vitro = glass). |
| Laparoscopy | A surgical procedure used to view abdominal organs such as the ovaries and Fallopian tubes using an illuminated instrument known as a laparoscope. |
| Libido | Libido refers to the intensity of sexual desire. |

| | |
|---|---|
| Luteal phase | The post-ovulatory phase characterised by the growth and development of the corpus luteum. |
| Luteinising hormone (LH) | Hormone secreted by the anterior pituitary that stimulates ovulation in women and the secretion of testosterone by the testes in men. |
| Menarche | The first menstrual period signifying the beginning of a young girl's reproductive life. |
| Menopause | The last menstrual period a woman experiences at the end of her reproductive life. |
| Menstrual cycle | The recurring cycle of physiological changes that occurs in reproductive-age females. There are two phases to the menstrual cycle: the follicular phase (menstruation to ovulation) and the luteal phase (ovulation to menstruation). |
| Menstruation, menses, menstrual period | The cyclic shedding of the endometrium, consisting of blood, mucus and cellular debris. Menstruation normally occurs about two weeks after ovulation when fertilisation has not occurred. |
| Miscarriage or spontaneous abortion | The premature and spontaneous loss of the embryo or foetus from the uterus. |
| Mittelschmerz, or ovulation pain | One-sided sharp pain or dull ache in the lower abdomen occurring around the time of ovulation. |
| Oestrogen/s | Female hormones secreted by the ovaries that bring about the secondary sex characteristics and regulate the female reproductive cycle.<br><br>Increasing oestrogen levels in the follicular phase (pre-ovulatory phase) of the cycle stimulates significant changes in the cervix, cervical mucus, and the endometrium. |

| | |
|---|---|
| Ovarian Hyper Stimulation Syndrome (OHSS) | This can occur during fertility treatment if the woman is overstimulated resulting in a large number of follicles/eggs, causing abdominal bloating, pain, nausea and breathlessness. |
| Orgasm | The climax of sexual excitement in the male or female. |
| Ovary | The female reproductive organ which produce eggs and the female sex hormones oestrogen and progesterone. These hormones control the menstrual cycle and female secondary sex characteristics. |
| Ovulation | The process in which a mature egg/ovum is released from a follicle. |
| Polycystic Ovarian Syndrome (PCOS) | A condition where multiple, small follicles develop around the outside of the ovary. |
| Pituitary gland | The 'master' endocrine gland at the base of the brain which produces many important hormones, some of which trigger other glands into making their own hormones. The pituitary functions include hormonal control of the ovaries and testes. |
| Placenta | The placenta develops after implantation of an embryo. It provides nutrients to a developing foetus, carries away wastes, and produces hormones such as oestrogen and progesterone. |
| Post-ovulatory phase (luteal phase) | The phase from ovulation to the onset of the next menstruation. It has a relatively constant length, usually lasting from 12 to 16 days. |
| Premature ovarian failure (POF) | POF occurs when the ovaries stop working properly, usually due to loss or dysfunction of egg follicles. It can be reversible. |
| Premature menopause | Early onset of menopause resulting in an inability to conceive naturally. |

| | |
|---|---|
| Premenstrual syndrome | A collection of physical and emotional signs and symptoms which appear during the post-ovulatory phase and disappear at the onset of menstruation. |
| Pre-ovulatory phase | The variable-length phase from the onset of menstruation to ovulation. |
| Progesterone | Female hormone secreted by the ovaries which prepares the endometrium for a possible pregnancy. It is also responsible for the rise in basal body temperature, for changing the cervix to its infertile state and for changing the cervical mucus to form an impenetrable barrier to sperm. |
| Prolactin | A hormone secreted by the anterior pituitary which stimulates the production of breast milk and inhibits the ovarian production of oestrogen. |
| Puberty | The time of life in boys and girls when the reproductive organs become functional and the secondary sexual characteristics appear. |
| Seminal fluid or semen | The fluid ejaculated from the penis at orgasm. The viscous fluid contains sperm and secretions from the seminal vesicles and prostate gland. |
| Sperm / spermatozoon | The mature male sex cell. |
| Subfertility | A state of reduced fertility. |
| Testicle/testes | One of a pair of male sex glands which produces sperm and the male sex hormones or androgens including testosterone. |
| Testosterone | Male hormone secreted by the testes that stimulates the growth of the male reproductive organs and brings about the secondary sex characteristics. |
| Umbilical cord | Structure that connects the embryo/foetus to the placenta. |

| | |
|---|---|
| Ultrasound | A diagnostic technique which uses sound waves to produce an image of internal body structures. |
| Uterus | The pear-shaped muscular organ in which the fertilised embryo implants and grows for the duration of pregnancy. Also known as the womb. |
| Vasectomy | Male sterilisation operation in which the vas deferens is cut and the ends separated to prevent the passage of sperm. |
| Zygote | The fertilised ovum. A single fertilised cell resulting from fusion of the sperm and the egg cell. After further cell division the zygote is known as the embryo. |

## Bibliography

Allen, R.P. (2004) *Scripts and Strategies in Hypnotherapy*. Carmarthen: Crown House Publishing.

American Psychiatric Association (2000) *Diagnostic and statistical manual of mental disorders*, 4th edition, text revision. Washington, DC: American Psychiatric Association.

American Psychological Association (2000) *The American Heritage Dictionary of the English Language,* 4th edition. Boston: Houghton Mifflin.

Benedek, T. (1953) 'Some Emotional Factors in Infertility', *Psychosomatic Medicine*, 15 (5), 485–98.

Berland, W. (1998) *Out of the box for life.* New York: Harper Collins.

Blythe, P. (1976) *Self Hypnotism.* London: Arthur Baker.

Bryant, P.M. (2006) *Hypnotherapy for Dummies*. Chichester, West Sussex: John Wiley and Sons.

Chopra, D. (1994) *Ageless Body, Timeless Mind.* New York: Harmony.

Chopra, D. (2000) *Magical Mind Magical Body*. Niles: Nightingale Conant (Audiobook)

De Shazer, S. (1985) *Keys to Solution in Brief Therapy.* New York: Norton.

Dick-Read, D.G. (2005) *Childbirth without Fear: The Principles and Practice of Natural Childbirth* 4th edition. London: Pinter and Martin Ltd.

Dilts, R. (1980) *Neurolinguistic Programming Volume 1.* Capitola: Meta Publications.

Dilts, R. and DeLozier, J. (2000) *Encyclopedia of systemic NLP and NLP New Coding.* Scotts Valley: NLP University Press.

Dispenza, J. (2007) *Evolve your brain: the science behind changing your mind.* Deerfield Beach: Health Communications.

Domar, A. (n.d.) *Infertility and Stress*. Retrieved 2007 from www.bostonivf.com: www.bostonivf.com/mind_body_center/InfertilityandStress.pdf.

Domar, A. et al (1992) 'The Prevalence and Predictability of Depression in Infertile Woman', *Fertility and Sterility, 58*, 1158–63.

Domar, A. and Kelly, A. (2002) *Conquering Infertility: Dr Alice Domar's guide to enhancing fertility and coping with infertility.* London: Viking Penguin.

Eastburn, L. (2006) *It's conceivable!* Victoria, Canada: Trafford Publishing.

Erickson, M. and Rossi, E. (1976) 'Two-Level Communication and the Microdynamics of Trance and Suggestion', *The American Journal of Clinical Hypnosis, 1.*

Facchinetti, F. et al (1997) 'An increased vulnerability to stress is associated with a poor outcome of in vitro fertilisation – Embryo transfer treatment'. *Fertility and Sterility, 67,* 309-14.

*Fertility UK Glossary* (2009, January). Retrieved from http://www.fertilityuk.org/: http://www.fertilityuk.org/nfps02.html#glossaryovulationmethod.

Greaves, S. (2002) 'Can hypnosis help to make you pregnant?', *The Times.* Retrieved 6 July 2008, from http://www.timesonline.com.

Griffin, J. and Tyrrell, I. (2004a) *How to lift depression fast.* Chalvington: HG Publishing.

Griffin, J. and Tyrrell, I. (2007) *How to master anxiety.* Chalvington: HG Publishing.

Griffin, J. and Tyrrell, I. (2004b) *Human Givens: A new approach to emotional health and clear thinking.* Chalvington: HG Publishing.

Grille, R. (2008) *Heart to Heart Parenting.* Ultimo: ABC Books.

Hammond, D.C. (1990) *Handbook of hypnotic suggestions and metaphors.* New York: W.W. Norton and Company.

HFEA (2008) *The HFEA guide to Infertility.* London.

Houser, P.M. (2007) *Fathers-To-Be Handbook: A Road Map for the Transition to Fatherhood.* Lamberhurst: Creative Life Systems.

Hunter, R. (2005) *Hypnosis for Inner Conflict Resolution: Introducing Parts Therapy.* Carmarthen: Crown House Publishing.

Indichova, J. (2002) '3 Steps Forward'. On *Fertile Heart Imagery* [CD]. New York: Julia Indichova.

*Infertility Glossary* (2009). Retrieved February 2009 from Georgia Reproductive Specialists: http://www.ivf.com/gloss.html.

Jeker, et al. (1988) 'Wish for a child and infertility', *International Journal of Fertility*, 33 (6), 411–20.

Kluger-Bell, K. (1998) *Unspeakable losses: Healing from Miscarriage, Abortion, and Other Pregnancy Losses.* New York: W.W. Norton and Company.

Kübler-Ross, E. (2005) *On Grief and Grieving: Finding the Meaning of Grief Through the Five Stages of Loss.* Princeton: Scribner.

Levitas, E. (2006) 'Impact of hypnosis during embryo transfer on the outcome of in vitro fertilization-embryo transfer: a case-control study', *Fertility and Sterility*, 85 (5), 1404–08.

Lewis, R.P. (2004) *The Infertility Cure.* New York: Little, Brown and Company.

Lipton, D.B. (2005) *The Biology of Belief.* Santa Rosa: Mountain of Love/Elite Books.

Lockwood, G., Anthony-Ackery, J., Meyers-Thompson, J. and Perkins, S. (2007) *Fertility and Infertility for Dummies.* Chichester: John Wiley and Sons.

MedicineNet.com (2003) *Webster's New World Medical Dictionary*, 2nd edition. Springfield: Webster's New World.

Meldrum, D.R. (1993) 'Reproductive aging—ovarian and uterine factors',. *Fertility and Sterility*, 59, 1–5.

Nejad, L. and Volny, K. (2008) *Treating stress and anxiety.* Carmarthen: Crown House Publishing.

NHS (2008) *Patient information leaflet – Miscarriage.* Retrieved 12 August 2008, from NHS – National Library for Health: http://cks.library.nhs.uk/patient_information_leaflet/miscarriage.

Nicholas, M. (2006) *3 Steps to fertility.* London: Carroll and Brown Publishers Limited.

Northrup, Christiane (1998) *Women's Bodies, Women's Wisdom: The Complete Guide to Women's Health and Wellbeing*, 2nd revised edition. London: Piatkus Books.

Pascual-Leone, D., et al (1995) 'Modulation of muscle response evoked by the transcranial magnetic stimulation during the aquisition of new fine motor skills', *Journal of Neurophysiology*, 74 (3), 1037–45.

Payne, N.B. (1997) *The whole person fertility programme: A revolutionary mind-body process to help you conceive.* New York: Three Rivers Press.

Payne, N. and Richardson, B. (2002) *The Fertility Solution: A reveloutionary mind-body process to help you conceive.* London: Thornsons.

Pert, C. (1999) *Molecules of Emotion: Why You Feel the Way You Feel.* New York: Touchstone.

Pert, C. (1985) 'Neuropeptides and their receptors: A psychosomatic network', *Journal of Immunology* (2), 135.

Petty, R.G. (2007) 'Healing, Meaning and Purpose: The Magical Power of the Emerging Laws of Life', iUniverse.com.

Pope, A. (2001a) *The Wild Genie: the healing power of menstruation.* Bowral, Australia: Sally Milner Publishing.

Pope, A. (2001b) *Walking with the Genie: The Modern Woman's Menstrual Health Kit.* Self-Published.

Quinn, P. and Pawson, M. (1994) 'Psychosomatic Infertility', *European Journal of Clinical Hypnosis*, 4, 1–10.

Rossi, E.L. (2002) *The Psychobiology of Gene Expression: Neuroscience and neurogenesis in hypnosis and the healing arts.* New York: W.W. Norton and Company Ltd.

Rossi, E.L. and Cheek, D.B. (1994) *Mind-Body Therapy; ideodynamic healing in hypnosis.* New York: W.W. Norton.

Schwartz, J. (2008) *The mind-body fertility connection: The true pathway to conception.* Woodbury: Llewellyn Publications.

Shapiro, D. (2008) *Your body speaks your mind.* London: Piakatus Books.

Simpkins C.A. and Simpkins A.M. (2004) *Self Hypnosis For Women*. San Diego: Radiant Dolphin Press.

Singer, K. (2004) *The Garden of Fertility: A Guide to Charting Your Fertility Signals to Prevent or Achieve Pregnancy—Naturally—and to Gauge Your Reproductive Health*. New York: Avery.

Tan, S. et al (1992) 'Cumulative conception and livebirth rates after in-vitro fertilisation', *The Lancet*, 339 (8806), 1390–94.

Waxman, D. (1998) *Medical and Dental Hypnosis*. Bath: Bookcraft.

Wilson, R.A (1990) *Quantum Psychology: How Brain Software Programmes You and Your World*. Tempe: New Falcon Publications.

Wolinsky, S. (1991) *Trances People Live: Healing approaches in quantum psychology*. Las Vegas: The Bramble Company.

Wood, C.C. (1992) 'Age and fertility: results of assisted reproductive technology in women over 40 years', *Journal of Assisted Reproduction and Genetics*, 9 (5), 482–4.

# *Index*

10 to 1 Self-Hypnosis 181, 184, 282

7:11 Breathing 68, 71, 73, 146, 163, 181, 183, 280, 290, 324, 325, 340

Abnormal Ovulation 16

Abortions 106, 113, 284, 355, 363, 368, 375

Adoption 170, 171, 172, 296, 299, 300, 357

Adrenaline 59, 62, 67, 120

Affirmations 74, 77, 140, 146, 161, 185, 279, 283, 284, 327

Age 19, 23, 46, 57, 67, 89, 91, 103, 104, 106, 108, 116, 147, 150, 320, 368, 377

Amenorrhoea 116, 363

Anchors 88, 154, 160, 181, 216, 218

Androgens 17, 363, 370

Anovulation 16, 50, 67, 80, 116, 330, 363

Anxiety 7, 12, 19, 28, 50, 55, 57, 59, 60, 62, 67, 69, 70, 73, 74, 77, 103, 109, 110, 114, 115, 130, 138–42, 145, 146, 163, 164, 168, 177, 178, 200, 221–3, 282, 293, 294, 298, 309, 319, 320, 326, 327, 332, 334, 335, 337, 340, 342, 345, 346, 348, 356, 359, 374, 375

Apposition Of Opposites 63, 65, 76, 81, 123, 135, 181, 218, 326, 327, 336, 339, 347, 349

Assisted Conception Unit (ACU) 363

Assisted Reproductive Technology (ART) 67, 154, 296, 298, 309, 363, 377

Autonomic Nervous System (ANS) 57, 73, 290, 363

Basal body temperature (BBT) 20, 51, 303, 305, 363, 370

Beliefs 12, 15, 16, 23, 53, 55–7, 59–62, 68, 72, 74, 75, 85, 86, 93, 95–8, 105–7, 109, 110, 112, 124, 140, 146, 166, 173, 176, 179, 190, 193, 196, 197, 203, 219, 221, 232, 263, 283, 292, 294, 301, 327–9, 332, 337, 343

Beliefs 93, 95–7, 192, 197, 332

Biological rhythms 119

Bird Cage Release 102, 107, 112, 165, 170, 182, 246

Birth 4, 6, 23, 27, 29, 35, 47, 48, 57, 90–3, 96, 98, 101, 113, 115, 137, 140, 143–8, 163, 189, 190, 197, 213, 214, 226, 230, 246, 248, 249, 256, 269, 271, 293, 296, 299, 300, 314, 322, 323, 326, 327, 355, 358, 360, 366

Birth trauma 6, 35, 96, 143, 163

Blastocyst 277, 307, 308, 363

Body Talk 81, 102, 122, 129, 134, 181, 239, 339

Breathing Colour 68, 71, 73, 85, 177, 181, 186, 267, 324, 336

Case History 26, 46, 47, 52, 82, 95, 117, 163, 164, 166, 324

Case study 23, 25, 26, 49, 52, 53, 82, 84, 90, 131, 133, 134, 137, 139, 141, 147, 152, 273, 298, 311, 330, 335, 344, 346

Cellular Memory Recall 102, 104, 123, 140, 182, 248

Ceremony 107, 111, 165, 167, 170, 174, 279, 284, 328, 329

Cervical mucus 17, 20, 21, 302, 303, 305, 314, 364, 368, 370

Cervix 18, 21, 108, 109, 144, 145, 260, 275, 302, 303, 305, 313, 333, 363, 364, 368, 370

Cognitive Behavioural Therapy 61

Cognitive Restructuring 76-78, 97, 102, 103, 124, 166, 171, 173, 280, 292, 328, 329, 337, 343, 346

Complete miscarriage 109

Conception ii, 1, 2, 4, 6, 13, 14, 17, 50, 62, 64, 65, 70, 91–3, 98, 115, 118, 129, 132, 138, 142, 182, 212, 213, 248–50, 257, 276, 296–8, 301, 306–8, 312, 317, 319, 322, 325, 326, 341, 342, 349, 354, 360, 361, 363–7, 376

Connect With Your Inner Body 81, 121, 182, 259

Conscious Mind 11, 50, 213

Control Room 80, 83, 123, 132, 181, 200, 201, 318, 326, 336, 339, 340, 349

Corpus luteum (yellow body) 303, 304, 364, 368

Cortisol 62, 364

Create balance 55, 58, 60, 62, 76, 197

Creating A Fertile Body 102, 132, 182, 256, 336

Creative Tasks 121, 122, 141, 175, 279, 287, 337, 341–3

Cues 47, 77, 148, 159, 217, 231, 283, 343

Curettage/D and C 364

Current medical treatments available 296, 309

Damaged Fallopian tubes 17, 316

Damaged sperm ducts 18

Depression 7, 16, 36, 55, 60, 63, 69–71, 77, 92, 152, 193, 195, 319, 320, 327, 356, 358, 359, 374

Diet 4, 6, 53–7, 63, 64, 135, 358

Dilated veins around the testicle 18

Doors Of Perception 65, 76, 104, 107, 124, 171, 181, 192, 328, 331

Down regulation 332–3, 364

Dysmenorrhoea 116, 364

Dyspareunia 364

Ectopic pregnancy 17, 46, 365

Egg 16–18, 51, 56, 82, 95, 103, 116, 129, 153, 172, 177, 264–6, 274–6, 277, 297–9, 302, 305–9, 312, 314–8, 320–2, 325, 326, 333, 337–40, 342, 348, 349, 363–7, 369, 371

Egg collection 333, 337, 339, 340, 348

Egg donation 172, 322

## Index

Embryo 129, 132, 182, 264–71, 276–8, 297, 307, 309, 312, 314, 317, 320, 321, 325, 326, 333, 334, 340–3, 348–9, 363, 365, 367, 368–71, 374, 375

Embryo donation 297, 309, 312, 325, 348

Embryo transfer (ET) 129, 132, 182, 265, 267, 268, 270, 320, 321, 325, 333, 340, 341, 374, 375

Emotional Bank Account 83, 161, 280, 291, 329

Emotional needs audit 71–2

Emotional states 55, 66

Endometriosis 17, 21, 56, 64, 79, 80, 129, 131, 240, 312, 365

Endometrium 17, 21, 302, 303, 364, 365, 367, 368, 370

Enhance fertility I, 4, 7, 23, 27, 62, 80, 91, 127–9, 130, 133, 134, 190, 191, 219, 244, 254, 257, 263, 276

Exercise 6, 20, 53, 54, 63, 65, 68, 161, 327

External factors affecting fertility 19

Factors affecting the fertile state 55, 56, 98

Fallopian tube 21, 277, 302, 303, 307, 308, 317, 365

Fast Phobia Cure 96

Fatherhood 152, 179, 222, 355, 374

Fear Release 102, 124, 139, 145, 181, 224

Fertile phase 365

Fertile time 14, 51, 178, 296, 297, 305

Fertilisation 14, 129, 297, 303, 307, 312, 316, 317, 358, 363, 365–8, 374, 376

Fertility Awareness Education 20, 49, 50, 51, 301, 305

Fertility drugs 298, 311–3, 315, 316, 322, 323, 326, 330, 348

Fertility Garden 102, 106, 126, 132, 182, 263–4, 326, 328, 341

Fibroids 129, 134–5, 239, 240, 312

Fight-or-Flight response 9, 11, 57, 61, 73, 144

Finding meaning/Finding purpose 157, 173, 174

*Flare-up cycle* 333

Foetus 67, 90, 108, 307, 308, 365, 366, 368–70

Follicle 56, 79, 80, 244, 302, 304, 306, 364, 366, 369

Follicle stimulating hormone (FSH) 56, 80, 244, 302, 304, 306, 366

Follicular phase 301, 302, 304, 366, 368

Fostering 296, 300, 358

Free Floating Pseudo-orientation 83, 88, 182, 231

Free Floating Regression 101, 181, 208

Future Pacing 83, 132, 139, 151, 160, 170, 172, 182, 208, 229, 327, 329, 336, 343

Gamete intra-Fallopian transfer (GIFT) 298, 312, 317, 366

General health 19, 32, 55, 63

Goal setting 25, 27, 46, 82, 130, 133, 191, 323, 324, 344

Gonadotrophin-releasing hormone (GnRh) 306

Gonads 366

GP Diagnosis 46

Gratitudes 167, 279, 289, 343

Grief 6, 7, 108–12, 114, 118, 119, 167, 170, 251, 355, 375

Grief Ceremony/Ceremony To Say Goodbye 165, 167, 170, 174, 279, 284, 328, 329

Guided imagery 4, 125, 126, 128–30, 132, 133, 244

Healing Green Light 132, 182, 254, 324, 342

Healing White Light 81, 106, 107, 119, 126, 132, 134, 170, 182, 251, 328, 331, 339, 344, 345

Hormonal balance 50, 56, 70, 79, 81, 82, 116, 218, 244, 259, 261

Hormone deficiency 19

Hostile cervical mucus 17, 314

Human chorionic gonadotrophin (HCG) 367

Human development 296, 306

Human Fertilisation and Embryology Authority (HFEA) 14, 15, 319, 353, 358, 366, 374

Human Givens 58, 70–2, 208, 356, 358, 359, 374

Hypnotherapy and IVF 296

Hypothalamus 62, 67

Hypothalamus Meditation 68, 71, 73, 81, 123, 181, 244

Hysterosalpingogram (HSG) 366

Identify issues 54, 91, 95

Idiopathic infertility 367

Idiopathic low sperm count 18

Implantation 67, 79, 129, 132, 182, 268, 270, 303, 306, 308, 314, 316, 326, 333, 334, 340, 341, 365, 367, 369

Impotence 19, 314

IMR Signals – to locate past event 94, 97, 99, 100–2, 124, 134, 181, 210, 211, 214, 231

Incomplete miscarriage 109

Inevitable miscarriage 109

Infertility i–iii, 1, 6, 7, 13–18, 20, 52, 58, 69, 70, 75, 94, 106, 116, 123, 147, 157, 162, 170, 175, 281, 298, 312, 314, 316–20, 353, 354, 357, 359, 367, 373–6

Infradian rhythm 120

Inner conflict 23, 65, 86, 91, 97, 98, 101, 102, 105, 124, 172, 202, 204, 249, 374

Inner Emptiness Reintegration 170, 174, 181, 236

Inner Guide 81, 88, 110, 132, 133, 140, 167, 169, 182, 227, 228, 326, 328, 336, 341, 342

Inner resources 4, 5, 7, 35, 55, 56, 62, 72, 86, 90, 100, 101, 112, 114, 138, 139, 142, 154, 167, 205, 209, 217, 227, 298, 318, 324, 327-329, 332, 334–6, 341, 342, 345, 347

Intra-cytoplasmic sperm injection (ICSI) 177, 298, 312, 313, 316, 323, 363, 367

Intra-uterine insemination (IUI) (intra-cervical insemination (ICI)) 311

IVF Preparation 133, 182, 264, 332, 336, 339

In vitro fertilisation (IVF) 2, 4–6, 16, 70, 79, 86, 129, 130, 133, 137, 152, 154, 157, 165, 166, 177, 178, 182, 197, 200, 217, 246, 264, 265, 268, 270, 277, 296, 298, 299, 309, 312–4, 316, 317, 319–322, 332, 334–9, 341, 344–346, 348, 349, 363, 366, 367, 373–6

Laparoscopy 21, 367

Libido 51, 178, 367

Lifestyle 4, 15, 38, 53–5, 57, 63–5, 80, 84, 178, 306, 332, 335

Limiting beliefs 93, 95–7, 192, 197, 332

*Long protocol* 332

Low sperm count 18, 56, 70, 79, 80, 200, 316, 317

Luteal phase 301, 303, 304, 368, 369

Maintain Change 74, 157, 158–60, 227, 279

Male fertility 177

Male reproductive system 296, 306

Meditation 134, 169, 279, 285, 343, 360

Menarche 361, 368

Menopause 19, 103, 315, 357, 361, 368, 369

Menorrhagia 116

Menstrual Diary 280, 289

Menstrual Health 6, 23, 80, 89, 91, 96, 115, 116, 120, 236, 260–2, 301, 354, 361, 376

Menstruation 16, 20, 96, 116–9, 121, 122, 235, 243, 301–4, 354, 363–5, 368–70, 376

Mental Rehearsal 4, 12, 65, 72, 85, 88, 115, 125–130, 132, 134, 145, 148, 160, 163, 182, 229, 279, 286, 323, 325

Mindfulness 68, 71, 73, 163, 279, 282

Mini-Break Anchor 68, 71, 73, 140, 146, 164, 279, 282, 325, 343

Miscarriage 4–6, 14, 46, 64, 89, 91, 96–8, 105–14, 129, 138, 139, 141–2, 157, 163–5, 223, 246, 284, 313, 315, 326, 327, 332, 335, 360, 361, 364, 368, 375

Missed miscarriage 109

Modifying thought patterns 79

Moving on 24, 157, 170, 173–75

Natural conception ii, 13, 62, 91, 132, 277, 196–8, 301, 312, 322, 361

Needle phobia 96, 332

Neonatal death 23, 89, 91, 98, 114, 360

Nurturing 68, 121, 150, 163, 167, 255, 258, 266–9, 280, 291, 329, 337, 339, 341

Oestradiol 80

Oligomenorrhoea 116

Options for parenthood 7, 24, 157, 171, 297

Orange Dots 279, 283, 325, 343

Out Of The Box 233, 373

Ovarian Hyper Stimulation Syndrome (OHSS) 369

Ovarian Stimulation 317, 333

Ovaries 17, 21, 68, 82, 83, 104, 116, 191, 257, 259, 260, 264–6, 302, 315–7, 333, 338, 339, 363–70

Ovulation 16, 17, 20, 51, 67, 118, 119, 123, 297, 301-5, 312, 313, 330, 363, 364, 368–370

Ovulation predictor kits 305

Parts Work 65, 71, 77, 88, 94, 97, 100, 101, 104, 106, 107, 124, 153, 154, 169, 171, 172, 174, 182, 202–5, 298, 328, 344–6, 374

Pelvic inflammatory disease (PID)17

Physical symptoms 56, 79, 80, 120, 122, 133, 361

Pituitary gland 16, 67, 82, 244, 260, 302, 306, 366, 369

Placenta 64, 271, 277, 307, 308, 309, 369, 370

Polarity Exercise 151, 174, 178, 181, 221, 280, 294

Poor sperm morphology 18, 125, 129, 240

Pregnancy 2, 4–6, 17, 23, 29, 46, 51, 70, 79, 90, 91, 93, 97, 98, 101, 105–15, 130, 137, 138–43, 145, 146, 148, 157, 163, 164, 189, 197, 213, 224, 246, 248, 249, 269, 273, 285, 307, 312, 314, 316, 319, 320, 323, 326, 327, 333, 342, 346, 353–5, 358, 360, 361, 363–71, 375, 376

Premature menopause 357, 369

Premature ovarian failure (POF) 16, 359, 369

Premenstrual Syndrome (PMS) 121

Primal Image 73, 80, 83, 104, 111, 119, 126, 131, 132, 134, 140, 143, 177, 181, 190–1, 264, 326, 327, 339, 341, 349

*Primary infertility* 14

Progesterone 20, 67, 80, 302–4, 333, 364, 369, 370

Prolactin 16, 67, 370

Pseudo-orientation 72, 83, 88, 132, 138, 139, 145, 148, 151, 153, 160, 170, 172, 182, 202, 204, 213, 216, 229, 230, 231, 327, 329, 336, 342, 343

Puberty 119, 370

Questionnaire ii, 26, 38–45, 46–51, 324, 334

Quick Body Scan 68, 71, 73, 121, 162, 163, 280, 290, 339

Rape 97, 98

Reframing 206, 210

Relationship issues 4, 56, 84

Resource building 134, 138, 154, 212, 229, 234, 339

Resource Gathering 68, 72, 73, 83, 88, 122, 139, 142, 145, 151, 154, 167, 171, 181, 194, 205, 231, 323, 328, 336, 342, 346

Retrograde ejaculation 19, 22

Rewind Technique 96, 107, 147, 148, 181, 206, 210

Rituals 284, 285, 338, 339

Safe Place/Favourite Place 68, 83, 88, 112, 132, 145, 147, 148, 164, 181, 188, 189, 209, 266

Saliva tests 305

Scaling questions 35, 88

Scripts 181–278

*Secondary infertility* 14

Self-help tools 279–294

Self-Hypnosis 68, 69, 71, 73, 77, 121, 128, 132, 133, 135, 139, 140, 145, 146, 147, 160, 161, 163, 167, 172, 181, 184, 185, 187–9, 240, 247, 279, 281, 282, 290, 322, 325, 326, 329, 331, 337, 339, 340, 341, 348

Self-Integration Dissociation 63, 65, 88, 90, 95, 102, 104, 107, 121, 152, 154, 165, 167, 170, 174, 181, 187, 196, 327, 328, 336, 342, 347

Self-Talk SUDS 78, 140, 142, 280, 293, 329

Self-talk 4, 75, 77–9, 140, 142, 280, 293, 329

Seminal fluid (semen) 18, 19, 21, 22, 363, 365, 370

Sexual abuse 97, 98

Sexual performance problems 97

Sexual problems 99, 314

*Short protocol* 333

SMART goal 27–9

Solution Focused Therapy (SFT) 25, 30, 31, 347

Somatic Bridge Regression 101, 181, 214

Sperm antibodies 19

Sperm collection 333

Sperm donation 178

Spiritual beliefs 56, 85, 86

Stage 1: Outcome 5, 23, 25, 48, 55, 89, 90, 96, 130, 131, 133, 134, 141, 147, 191, 229, 231, 243, 257, 345

Stage 2: Balance 5, 16, 23, 29, 53, 55, 58, 86, 89, 90, 93, 96, 101, 112, 128, 130, 131, 133–5, 138, 142, 147, 152, 189, 193, 195, 197, 200, 203, 212, 217, 219, 221, 223, 227, 229, 231, 234, 244, 251, 260, 262, 330, 342, 345

Stage 3: Resolve 5, 23, 54, 55, 62, 75, 80, 86, 89, 134, 138, 142, 143, 147, 164, 189, 193, 195, 197, 203, 204, 207, 212, 222, 223, 225, 227, 234, 236, 237, 243, 246, 249, 251, 257, 260, 262, 263, 273, 301, 334

Stage 4: Enhance 23, 80, 89, 125, 130, 131, 133, 134, 135, 191, 219, 229, 234–57, 260, 263, 270, 274, 277

Stage 5: Prepare 23, 54, 89, 115, 124, 137, 143, 148, 163, 179, 197, 222, 229, 232, 246

Stage 6: Support 24, 54, 110, 115, 138, 148, 157, 193, 227, 236, 237

Stillbirth 6, 23, 24, 89, 91, 96, 98, 114, 157, 164, 284, 360

Storm Cloud Metaphor 174, 182

Stress 4, 6, 7, 9, 11, 16, 27–9, 49–51, 53, 55, 57, 61–3, 66–71, 77, 78, 81–6, 91, 99, 103, 117, 120, 121, 123, 134, 141, 144, 146, 158, 165, 177, 178, 187, 244, 292, 318, 321, 330, 332, 334–6, 344, 361, 364, 373–5

*Subfertility* 14, 370

Surgery 17–19, 131, 134, 189, 311, 312, 323, 326, 327, 333

Surrogacy 172, 296, 299, 312, 315, 325, 357

Termination of pregnancy 97, 273, 363

Terminations 4, 6, 89, 91, 98, 105, 106

Testicle (testes) 18, 363, 366, 368–70

Testosterone 17, 129, 64, 80, 177, 274, 306, 368, 370

The 3 Session Plan For ART 296, 309, 322, 323, 330

The 4 Session Plan For IVF 79, 296, 309, 322, 323, 334, 335, 346, 348

The Big Race 81, 132, 177, 182, 274

The Complete Plan For IVF 296, 309, 323, 346, 348

The effect of stress on fertility 67

The menstrual cycle 17, 20, 50, 51, 67, 81, 115, 116, 118–21, 123, 259, 296, 301, 302, 304, 361, 365, 368, 369

The mind-body connection 26, 49, 50

The Mirror Of Forgiveness 90, 95, 107, 182, 272–3

The stages of an IVF cycle 296, 309, 332

The two week wait 79, 129, 333, 334, 341, 342

Therapeutic strategy 25, 35, 47, 49

Threatened miscarriage 108

Three Steps Forward 115, 139, 140, 163, 181, 223, 224, 326

Treatment plan 5, 25, 26, 48, 52, 53, 86, 165, 309, 334, 346

Tune Into Your Body Clock 63, 123, 182, 261

Two stage dissociation 96

Ultradian rhythm 120

Ultrasound 21, 314, 371

Umbilical cord 269, 271, 370

Unconscious blocks 23, 55, 75, 89, 91, 93, 96, 99, 100, 102

Unconscious Mind 4, 10–12, 30, 50, 93, 96, 99–101, 122, 125, 129, 149, 190, 198, 199, 205, 208, 211–16, 230, 247, 260, 265–7, 287, 327

*Unexplained infertility* 14, 52, 106, 147, 298, 314, 316-318

Unhealthy beliefs 12, 53, 55, 57, 59–61, 75, 93, 97, 107, 110, 124, 166, 179, 193, 203, 221, 232, 294, 328, 329, 337, 343

Unresolved issues 4, 6, 75, 89–91, 93, 94, 96, 97, 102, 121, 203

Vasectomy 19, 312, 315, 371

Visualisation 1, 4, 6, 10, 11, 13, 21, 23, 50, 53, 80, 83, 90, 96, 110, 115, 121, 125–35, 139, 140, 145, 147, 151, 185, 186, 188, 196, 196, 223, 227, 246, 251, 254, 256, 259, 261, 263, 264, 267, 270, 272, 274, 276, 281, 283, 286, 306, 317, 322, 323, 325–7, 331, 335, 337–43, 349

Word Association 181, 243

Working with men iv, 23, 24, 177

Working with scales 35, 72, 139

Worry 50, 53, 63, 72–5, 77–9, 117, 122, 129, 130, 158, 163, 178, 335, 342, 343

Zygote 277, 307, 308, 316, 371

## *Acknowledgements*

I would like to thank the following people:

Lisa Jackson for kindly offering her time to help edit this book.
Verity Lewis, for your thoughts, ideas and helpful feedback which really helped me in the early days of writing this book.
My teacher and friend, Maggie Chapman, without whom I would not be a hynotherapist. Her wisdom is in the bones of this book.
Natalia O'Sullivan, for her insight into the ancestral aspects of fertility. Thank you for teaching me how to see what is in front of me.
Ya'acov Darling Khan, for encouraging me to keep paying attention. His teachings are in the heart of this book.
All the men and women I have worked with who have allowed me to learn and understand a little bit more about what it means to be human.
All of my students, who have inspired me, challenged me and taught me.
Mom and Dad, for giving me such a great start in life.
My husband Philip, for helping me to keep my sense of humour. Life is so joyful with you.